Pediatric Pain Management

Clinical Child Psychology Library

Series Editors: Michael C. Roberts and Annette M. La Greca

A Continuation Order Plan is available for this series. A continuation order will bring delivery of each new volume immediately upon publication. Volumes are billed only upon actual shipment. For further information please contact the publisher.

Pediatric Pain Management

Lynnda M. Dahlquist

University of Maryland, Baltimore County
Baltimore, Maryland

Kluwer Academic / Plenum Publishers
New York, Boston, Dordrecht, London, Moscow

Library of Congress Cataloging-in-Publication Data

Dahlquist, Lynnda M.
    Pediatric pain management / Lynnda M. Dahlquist.
        p.   cm. -- (Clinical child psychology library)
    Includes bibliographical references and index.
    ISBN 0-306-46084-X (hardbound). -- ISBN 0-306-46085-8 (pbk.)
    1. Pain in children--Treatment.   I. Title.   II. Series.
    [DNLM: 1. Pain--in infancy & childhood.   2. Pain--therapy.
3. Pain--etiology.   4. Pain Measurement--in infancy & childhood.
5. Cognitive Therapy--in infancy & childhood.   6. Patient Care
Planning.   WL 704 D131p 1999]
    RJ365.D34   1999
    616'.0472'083--dc21
    DNLM/DLC
    for Library of Congress   98-43928
                                                                         CIP

ISBN 0-306-46084-X (Hardbound)
ISBN 0-306-46085-8 (Paperback)

© 1999 Kluwer Academic / Plenum Publishers, New York
233 Spring Street, New York, N.Y. 10013

10 9 8 7 6 5 4 3 2 1

A C.I.P. record for this book is available from the Library of Congress.

Printed in the United States of America

Preface

Pain is a complex, multidimensional phenomenon, with physiological, behavioral, emotional, cognitive, and developmental aspects (Zeltzer, Barr, McGrath, & Schechter, 1992). To effectively evaluate and manage pain in children, the clinician must be able to assess the unique ways these complex dimensions interact for the individual child and integrate these dimensions into a treatment plan. This can be a daunting task.

The purpose of this book is to provide a framework for conceptualizing pain problems in children that can guide the practitioner in developing an evaluation and treatment plan that is optimal for the individual child. This book is not intended to be a comprehensive, exhaustive review of the literature on pain management in children. There are several excellent books of this nature (e.g., Bush & Harkins, 1991; McGrath, 1990; Ross & Ross, 1988). Instead, this book is an attempt to outline an hypothesis testing *process* of case conceptualizing and treatment planning that can help structure the task of sorting through the complex interrelationships that determine children's pain.

The recommendations presented herein are based on the childhood pain literature, my personal research experiences, and my clinical experiences treating pain problems in children. It is assumed that the reader already has some training and background in child development, clinical intervention with children and families, and basic cognitive therapy and behavior modification principles. Hence, the focus of this text is on the *unique* challenges faced in designing clinical interventions for pediatric pain problems.

I am indebted to Ted Wachs for teaching me early in my graduate career to think about psychotherapy as a scientist—to formulate hypotheses about my clients that are objective, testable, and based on the literature, to test my hypotheses in an objective fashion, and to formulate a treatment plan that is based on the resulting evidence and conceptualization. This hypothesis testing model serves as the foundation for the approach to pediatric pain management that is described in this book.

My personal research on pain management in children was greatly influenced by the supervision I received from Chuck Elliott and Susan Jay when I was an intern at Oklahoma University, and by their groundbreaking work in pain management in children. Their influence can be clearly seen in the cognitive–behavioral emphasis in the pain management strategies I have chosen to highlight in this text.

I would also like to acknowledge my psychology research collaborators, whose ideas and hard work contributed significantly to the ideas presented in this text—Jennifer Pendley, Tom Power, Donna Landthrip, and Cheri Jones. I also thank my many colleagues in pediatrics (particularly Don Fernbach, Phil Steuber, Chris Frantz, Bob Warren, Don Wuori, and the late Barbara Jones) for their sensitivity to pain problems in children and their willingness to collaborate on pediatric pain research. And last, but not least, I thank the many children and parents who participated in our clinical and research programs for sharing their concerns, their coping strategies, and their critiques of our efforts.

There are many additional people who deserve my heartfelt appreciation for their contributions to this project. First, I would like to thank Annette LaGreca and Mike Roberts for offering me this opportunity and for their constructive feedback on the text. I also thank my terrific team of graduate students for taking time out of their busy schedules to track down background materials for me and comment on drafts of the manuscript. I especially want to thank my friend and colleague, Danita Czyzewski, for her many hours of consultation and encouragement as I developed this book. Finally, I wish to thank my family—Carlo, Cara, and Anna—for their patience and love throughout this project.

Contents

Pediatric Pain Management

Introduction

A child in pain is one of the most compelling, as well as one of the most perplexing, clinical situations for most parents and health professionals. Few adults can remain untouched by the sobs or screams of a child in pain. Few parents can remain impervious to their child's pleas to "Make it better, Mommy!" or to the arms wrapped tightly around their neck as the child begs, "Don't let them hurt me." There is tremendous survival value to the gut-wrenching pull of a child in pain and the resulting human instinct to pay attention to the pain, to rescue the child, and make the pain go away. Yet, the same developmental qualities of young children that make them depend on adults for rescue and assistance also hamper adults' ability to help them with pain. Often, their language is not sophisticated enough to precisely communicate their experience of pain. This leaves the medical professional or parent the challenging job of trying to figure out what is wrong (or, in some cases leading adults to discount their experience entirely).

In addition, children seem primed to imitate pain symptoms, regardless of whether they actually are experiencing pain, and to use them to avoid unpleasant activities. For example, a 3-year-old can magically develop a "tummy ache" in order to avoid eating unpalatable vegetables. Thus, the challenge for the adults who care for children is to balance compassion and concern for the pain children experience, with the need to make sure that children do not inadvertently learn to use pain symptoms or disability to meet their emotional needs or solve their problems.

This challenge emerges regardless of whether the child's pain is acute (i.e., of short duration) or chronic (as in the case of protracted illnesses, recovery from injury or surgery, or painful conditions that last for years, such as arthritis). The purpose of this book is to provide a framework for conceptualizing and treating children's pain (regardless of the etiology of the pain) that addresses both objectives: the reduction of the pain experience and the minimizing of the negative consequences of pain behaviors (i.e., maximizing the developmentally appropriate functioning in children who experience pain). These guidelines are based on clinical and behavioral medicine research. However, the details and practical applications were developed in collaboration with the many children and parents encountered in our clinical practice and in our past and current research programs at the University of Maryland Children's Cancer Center, Johns Hopkins School of Medicine, Texas Children's Hospital and Baylor College of Medicine, and West Virginia University School of Medicine.

WHAT IS PAIN?

Years ago, pain was simply thought to be the body's response to injury or damage. The more tissue that was damaged, the more pain one would feel. Melzack and Wall (1965, 1982), in their now classic articles on the "gate control theory" of pain, effectively shattered this oversimplified conceptualization of pain. Pain is more than just a function of amount of injury. Different people with the same injury may have vastly different experiences of pain. Furthermore, a specific individual may experience widely ranging levels of pain depending on the situation. As Melzack and Wall noted, athletes may not even be aware of a serious injury during a heated competition, only to experience severe pain when the game is over. Emotional states, such as depression and anxiety, can exacerbate the experience of pain. In contrast, predictability and controllability of painful stimuli can lessen the perception of pain (Staub, Tursky, & Schwartz, 1971).

To explain these pain phenomena, Melzack and Wall proposed the existence of a gate-like mechanism that modulates whether physical pain sensations actually reach the brain to be perceived as pain. Pain sensations are transmitted to this gate in the dorsal horn of the spinal column. If the gate is "open," the impulse continues to the brain, where it is then recognized as pain. If the gate is "closed," no signal is transmitted to the brain and consequently no pain sensation is perceived. According to this theory, both sensory/physical processes and cognitive/emotional (central) processes are able to open or shut this gate. A very simplified version of their theory follows. (See Melzack [1993] or McGrath [1990] for more elaborate discussions of gate control theory and the presumed underlying physiological mechanisms.)

Pain sensations are carried on two types of nerve fibers. A-delta fibers are large-diameter myelinated neurons and are thought to transmit "first pain" sensations, "the immediate stinging, sharp and well localized pain sensation" that accompanies an injury such as stubbing a toe (McGrath, 1990, p. 97). The more diffuse, burning, less localized pain that follows 1–2 seconds later is related to C fibers, which are smaller-diameter, slower-transmitting unmyelinated neurons. "Second" pain tends to last longer than the initial noxious stimulus (McGrath, 1990, p. 97). Sensory nerve fibers, in contrast, are primarily large-diameter, myelinated, A-type fibers and therefore conduct signals quickly.

Both noxious and innocuous afferent nerve fibers transmit information to specialized dorsal horn cells in the spinal column, which serve as complex receiving and relay (or gating) stations to the spinal column and ultimately to the brain

stem, thalamus, and cortex. If the sensory nerve impulses reach the "gate" before a pain impulse, the connecting neuron is stimulated and therefore unreceptive to the impulse from the pain fiber. The "gate" closes, thus blocking the perception of pain.

According to Melzack and Wall, this phenomenon explains why rubbing an arm or leg after bumping into something makes it feel better. The rubbing stimulates sensory nerve fibers, which then close the gate. This is one of the mechanisms thought to explain the effectiveness of transcutaneous electrical nerve stimulation (TENS) for chronic pain. TENS units provide very low intensity electrical stimulation to the skin near an injury and this stimulation transmitted via large fibers blocks messages transmitted by pain fibers (McGrath, 1990).

Melzack and Wall proposed that central cognitive processes also could function in a descending fashion to close or open the gate and thus affect pain perception. The scientific literature supports this notion. For example, in laboratory studies, people consistently describe painful stimuli, such as shocks, as less painful under certain kinds of cognitive conditions than others. (Shock is often used in these studies because it allows one to administer exactly the same painful stimulus each time and to each individual.) For example, when a light signals the shock (i.e., when the shock is predictable), it is perceived as less painful than when presented without the signal. When individuals are told that they can adjust the intensity of the shock if it becomes unbearable (even if they never actually do any adjustments), they rate the pain as less unpleasant and habituate more rapidly to the shock than individuals who are not given the perception of control. Thus, the cognitive factors of perceived predictability and perceived control appear to moderate pain perception (Staub et al., 1971).

Distraction (diverting attention away from the pain stimulus) also influences pain perception. This is one of the principles behind natural childbirth techniques. The underlying assumption is that an individual has a finite attentional capacity and can only pay attention to a certain number of things at one time. The more attention that can be directed away from the pain experience, the less pain the person will experience (McCaul & Malott, 1984).

Anxiety and depression have been shown to increase rather than decrease pain perception, and according to Melzack and Wall's theory, open the gate. Thus, anything that counters anxiety and depression, such as muscle relaxation exercises or antidepressants, should close the gate and diminish pain perception.

Melzack and Wall's gate control model continues to influence current thinking about pain. Although some of the specific physiological mechanisms of the "gating" process proposed in the original model have been challenged (Melzack & Wall, 1982; Melzack, 1993), the fundamental components of this theory continue to guide conceptual models of pain. Therefore, any comprehensive understanding of pain must take into account the complex interaction of affective, cognitive, behavioral, and sensory–physical factors.

The experience of pain or the processes involved in pain perception are invisible to the observer. Pain occurs in the private internal experience of the individual. One infers pain experiences indirectly, from the grimaces, limping, groans, or words of the individual. In other words, one must rely on pain behaviors (either verbal or motor) to infer the pain experience of the individual. Thus, pain behavior comprises an additional component of the pain experience that is crucial to understand (Turk & Melzack, 1992). Pain behaviors and verbal descriptions of pain can provide the physician with extremely valuable information to assist in diagnosing the source of pain and in monitoring the effectiveness of pain relief efforts. For instance, throbbing head pain around the temples often indicates a vascular etiology, whereas head pain that gets worse when the patient bends over often indicates a sinus infection (Kunz & Finkel, 1987). The more precise the description of the pain, the more useful the information to the physician.

Clearly, children are at a big disadvantage in this respect. Lacking sophisticated language skills, they are unable to offer the precise descriptions of internal sensations often needed to diagnose their problems. This might result in delayed diagnoses, or in unfortunate scenarios, practitioners may not believe the child is actually in pain. The difficulty understanding a child's pain is further hampered by the fact that a variety of different emotional states may elicit what seem to be the same behavioral responses in a child. Crying for example, may reflect pain, fear, fatigue, anger, or all of the above! Although some parents may become very adept at distinguishing certain types of cries in their children, this task is virtually impossible for the health provider, and becomes nearly impossible even for the parent when a combination of factors is contributing to the child's distress.

This uncertainty about what is really wrong—what is making the child upset—makes parents uncertain about what they should do and ultimately inconsistent in their treatment of the child in pain. On the one hand, most parents recognize that they should not let children feign illness to "get away with something." Most parents would not knowingly let a child stay home from school if he or she clearly were not ill. But what should a parent do when he/she is uncertain? Most parents would feel horrible if they had told their child to "Go to school and quit trying to get out of the spelling test" and later discovered that the child actually had an ear infection. Such uncertainty (and, perhaps, guilt) often results in intermittent negative reinforcement of pain behaviors. Johnny learns that sometimes he doesn't have to dry dishes if he has a headache, and Jane learns to avoid spinach with a "tummy ache."

The same inconsistencies can emerge with respect to positive reinforcement of pain behaviors. How can one not cuddle and comfort a hurting child? Where should parents draw the line between nurturing and inadvertently reinforcing pain behavior? Again, the uncertainty adults experience in determining if a child is truly suffering makes this determination extremely difficult.

Evaluating Pain in Children

Before the clinician can provide optimally effective pain management, he/she must first develop a clear understanding of the factors contributing to an individual child's pain experience. This task is best conceptualized as an ongoing process of generating and testing hypotheses. As one accumulates evidence in support of certain hypotheses, a picture of the unique needs of the child and his/her family emerges, allowing the clinician to develop an individualized treatment plan.

The basic steps in this model were adapted from basic behavioral assessment principles (e.g., Watson & Gresham, 1998) and clinical psychology case conceptualization strategies and are outlined in Table 2.1.

The first step in the process is to develop a clear picture of the child's pain problem. The clinician should develop an operational definition of the problematic pain behaviors as well as the alternative adaptive behaviors that one hopes would replace the maladaptive pain behaviors. The description of the pain problem should include the physical, cognitive, emotional, and behavioral aspects of the child's pain responses as well as the conditions under which these responses occur.

The next step involves generating hypotheses regarding possible causes of the pain problem. These hypotheses should consider all possibilities, even unlikely ones, to avoid conducting a biased or incomplete evaluation. For each hypothesis, the clinician determines how the hypothesis could be tested. In other words, what data or evidence could be collected to support or refute each hypothesis, and how could that data be obtained? A list of possible sources of data is then generated for each hypothesis.

After a comprehensive listing of data sources is generated, the clinician prioritizes the assessment strategies in terms of the data sources that are likely to yield the most information and the most crucial information. This prioritized list serves as the assessment plan.

Table 2.1. The Steps in the Hypothesis Testing Approach to Pain Management

---

1. Describe the pain problem, including physical, cognitive/emotional, and behavioral components.
2. Generate hypotheses regarding possible causes of this problem.
3. Determine how each hypothesis could be tested.
4. Prioritize assessment strategies in terms of sources of data that are likely to yield the most critical information.
5. Conduct assessments to test each hypothesis.
6. Identify hypotheses supported and not supported by the data.
7. Plan treatment based on the data..
8. Evaluate treatment effectiveness.
9. If treatment outcome is less than optimal, return to # 2.
   Re-examine and refine hypotheses, add new hypotheses, conduct additional assessments as indicated by new or revised hypotheses, and update assessment findings.
10. Revise treatment plan.
11. Implement revised treatment plan.
12. Evaluate treatment effectiveness. (Go to # 9.)

The clinician then follows the assessment plan, keeping track of the resulting data and whether or not the data support or refute the proposed hypotheses. Once adequate data have been obtained, it should be possible to identify which of the hypotheses are supported and which hypotheses do not appear to be supported by the data. This serves as the working case conceptualization of the child's pain problem.

Designing the treatment plan is relatively straightforward at this point. The treatment plan should address each of the supported hypotheses. Treatment is then implemented according to the plan and the effectiveness of treatment is monitored.

If treatment is not effective, the hypothesis generation and testing process should be re-initiated. Possible hypotheses may have been omitted from the initial consideration, or new data may emerge that supports a different hypothesis. Additional data collection also may be needed. Based on the new evidence, the clinician identifies the hypotheses supported by the data and revises the conceptualization. The clinician then implements a revised treatment plan based on the empirically validated conceptualization. If the treatment is ineffective, the cycle of hypothesis generation and testing repeats.

It may be simplest to conceptualize this process in its entirety in the chart format presented in Figure 2.1. The clinician specifies the problematic pain behaviors in the left-hand column. Hypothesized causes are listed in the next column. To the right of each hypothesis, the clinician specifies the data needed to test the hypothesis. As data are collected, the clinician notes whether the findings support or refute the hypothesis. A treatment plan is designed to address each supported hypothesis. Finally, the clinician monitors treatment effectiveness.

Problematic pain behaviors	Hypothesized contributors to the child's pain	Potential sources of data to test hypotheses	Test results (yes, no, ?)	Treatment plan (based on test results)	Treatment evaluation

Figure 2.1. Brief overview of the hypothesis testing model for case conceptualization and treatment planning.

As can be seen in the overview of the various hypotheses presented in Figure 2.2, there are many important factors that should be considered in a comprehensive pain evaluation. A set of worksheets are provided in the Appendices that may be photocopied to help organize the processes of hypothesis generation and testing (Appendix A) and treatment planning and evaluation (Appendix B). These worksheets and the materials covered in the chapters that follow are not meant to be exhaustive. Rather, the intent is to provide guidelines and suggest important areas to investigate. The clinician should adapt these guidelines to each individual child and add and refine hypotheses as needed. Extra blank worksheets are provided for individualized hypotheses and treatment plans.

Hypothesized contributors to the child's pain	Potential sources of data	Test results	Treatment plan	Treatment evalualtion
Physical				
1. Is the child receiving less than optimal pain medication?	Parent interview	1.	1.	
Are available methods not being used?	Child interview			
2. Are medications administered inappropriately?	Medical staff interview	2.	2.	
Is the current dose inappropriate?	(MD, RN, therapist)			
Are medications administered at inappropriate times?	Chart review			
Are the medications scheduled inappropriately?	Medication records			
Are medications prescribed p.r.n.?	Observe child			
Is the child experiencing breakthrough pain?	Child pain diary			
3. Is the child failing to get all scheduled medication doses?	Parent pain records	3.	3.	
Is the child or family having problems with adherence?				
Are doses late or forgotten?				
Is the medication measured inaccurately?				
Are beliefs/misconceptions interfering?				
4. Are pain medications unavailable?		4.	4.	
Are finances preventing purchase of the medications?				
Is someone else using the medication?				
5. Are other physical factors exacerbating the child's pain?		5.	5.	
Is protective posturing or muscle tension causing additional discomfort or interfering with movement?				
Is fatigue interfering with pain coping efforts?				
Are environmental factors exacerbating pain?				
Is the child over-exerting, failing to use appropriate rest periods, or otherwise not following PT recommendations?				
Are other medications or other physical problems affecting his/her emotional, cognitive, or behavioral functioning?				

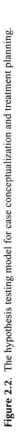

Cognitive and Emotional

1. Is the child's attention focused on the pain?
2. Is anxiety or stress exacerbating the child's pain?
   Are aspects of the child's environment frightening?
   Are clear signals for the onset and termination of painful stimuli lacking?
   Does the pain increase under stressful conditions?
3. Does the child engage in self-defeating thinking about the pain?
4. Does the pain have significant meaning for the child?
5. Is the caregiver's emotional or cognitive status interfering with his/her ability to assist the child in managing the pain?

Behavioral

1. To what degree is the child's pain behavior positively reinforced?
2. To what degree is the child's pain behavior negatively reinforced?
3. Is the child's adaptive behavior inadequately reinforced or punished?
4. Does the child lack the skills necessary to perform the adaptive behavior?
   Cognitive/academic deficits?
   Social/communication deficits?
5. To what degree is the adult's problematic behavior positively reinforced?
6. To what degree is the adult's problematic behavior negatively reinforced?
7. Is appropriate adult behavior inadequately reinforced or punished?

Cognitive and Emotional	
1. Child interview	1.
2. Parent interview	2.
Medical staff interview (MD, RN, therapist)	
Teacher interview	
3. Observe child	3.
4. Child pain diary	4.
5. Parent pain records	5.
Behavioral	
1. Interviews with: parent, child, medical staff, teachers	1.
2.	2.
3.	3.
4. Child pain diary	4.
Parent pain records	
Observe child	
5. Cognitive and academic testing	5.
6. Social functioning screening measures	6.
7.	7.

Figure 2.2. The hypothesis testing model for case conceptualization and treatment planning.

DEVELOPING AN OPERATIONAL DEFINITION
OF THE CHILD'S PAIN PROBLEM

Although this first stage of the model seems straightforward, obtaining a precise understanding and operational definition of the pain problem can be complicated. Basic behavioral assessment principles (e.g., Gelfand & Hartman, 1984; Martin & Pear, 1999; Mash & Terdal, 1988; Ollendick & Hersen, 1984) are helpful in guiding this stage of analysis. The resulting description of the child's pain problem should answer the following questions:

1	When does the child have pain? Under what conditions or in what settings?
2	What is the quality, frequency, intensity, and severity of the child's pain?
3	What are the behavioral, biological, and social consequences of the child's pain?

At this stage, as in each subsequent stage of the evaluation process, it is crucial to keep in mind that the various participants in the child's life may have very different impressions of the problem. Thus, although the therapist may be consulted by the physician or hired by the parents, it is important to assess perceptions of the pain problem at all three levels: the child, the family, and the medical/social system. We will consider each level separately.

THE CHILD'S PERSPECTIVE

A caveat is presented here before progressing to the actual content of pain assessment with children. The same factors that are essential to the development of rapport and the establishment of a therapeutic relationship also apply to pain management. Children need to know who the therapist is and what the therapist's role is. In the medical setting, it is especially important to reassure children that the therapist is a "talking" doctor or "pain specialist," and not someone who administers shots or causes other physical discomfort. Many children are afraid to report pain, fearing that they will get a "shot" or some other noxious treatment if they report symptoms. A few minutes of rapport building and discussion of nonthreatening topics help begin to establish a relationship with the child. Young children who are quite ill or have undergone traumatic, painful procedures may need several brief sessions before they will be able to discuss their painful experiences. Even if the child does not answer questions or volunteer information, by speaking directly to him/her the clinician communicates the important message that the child and his/her feelings are valued.

Pain assessment issues that emerge at different developmental levels are discussed in the following sections of this book. For a more detailed discussion of developmentally sensitive child interviewing techniques, see Hughes and Baker (1990).

Preschoolers

Before talking with a very young child, the clinician should consult the child's parents or nurse to determine the words the child uses to refer to pain. For instance, does he have an "owie" or a "boo-boo"? The clinician should then use the child's words whenever possible.

I typically offer the following reassurance before attempting to get any specific pain information from the child: "I promise I won't touch your 'owie.' Show me your 'owie.' Point to it." One should avoid the trap of asking yes/no questions in this and any assessment of a young child. Most yes/no questions (e.g., "Can you show me where it hurts?) are answered "No" by unhappy preschoolers, leaving the clinician with little choice but to badger the child into agreeing to show his "boo boo" after he has already declined (this approach rarely goes well), or to try again later.

Next, one should try to determine whether or not the child has a concept of relative magnitude by asking about the size of common objects in the environment. This can be done in a playful manner and can serve as part of rapport building. For example: "Let's think of something really small, really little. Name something really little. What about a mouse? Is a mouse little or big? Yes, a mouse is very little. What about a house? Is a house little or big? Yes, a house is very big..." Once the precision with which the child can rank concrete stimuli in terms of size has been established, the clinician can then use this ranking system to approximate the intensity of the child's pain. For example, one could ask: "Tell me about your 'boo boo' right now. Is it a big hurt or a little hurt?"

Up to the age of 4, it is difficult to get even simple intensity ratings of pain. This may reflect the difficulty the young child has considering multiple factors at the same time in order to consider relative dimensions. Many preschoolers describe their current emotional or physical states in rigid, simplified terms—either good or bad, pain or no pain. The current pain, be it a stubbed toe or a healing surgical incision, is bad if it exists, and not bad when it goes away. It is best not to push to get an intensity estimate if it is at all difficult for the child.

Early Elementary School Age

As children develop more knowledge of their bodies, they can begin to distinguish whether pain sensations are internal or on the surface skin. They can begin to evaluate relative pain intensity, but are likely to be more accurate in reporting current states than in retrospective recall of past experiences. Intensity ratings should be kept simple at this age. For example, with training, many 5- and 6-year-olds can use visual analog scales like the one presented below to indicate pain intensity (McGrath, 1990). The child is asked to make a mark bisecting the line to show how much he/she hurts. The distance from the left end point of the line to the child's mark is then measured and serves as the index of pain severity.

No pain   _____ Very bad pain

It is often a good idea first to test out the child's ability to use this sort of visual analog scale using another less abstract sensory dimension. Most elementary school-aged children understand the notion of food preferences and can use visual analog scaling to communicate their preferences.

How much do you like spinach?
    not at all   _____very much
How much do you like hot dogs?
    not at all   _____very much
How much do you like chocolate ice cream?
    not at all   _____very much

Late Elementary School Age

As children become increasingly able to ponder multiple events at the same time, it becomes possible to ask about past or hypothetical experiences. For example, the clinician can tell the child: "Think about a time when your pain was very bad and tell me about it." However, the veracity of these estimates still needs to be viewed cautiously. As is true of adults, children are often very bad at objectively analyzing their own experiences, especially retrospectively. What this line of assessment may provide, however, is an idea of certain events, thoughts, physical positions, or individuals that the child associates with pain.

Adolescents

Most of the measures of pain used with adults are compatible with the cognitive abilities of adolescents. For example, one can ask for pain intensity ratings on a scale of 0 to 100. Adolescents may be able to identify qualitative aspects of their pain that younger children cannot identify, such as searing versus throbbing versus stinging. (See Turk and Melzack [1992] for a comprehensive review of adult pain assessment strategies.) However, one should not just hand the adolescent a questionnaire and assume it will be completed in a careful, valid manner. The adolescent may not understand the measure, may not approach it in a serious manner, or may complete it carelessly. Although questionnaires may require less therapist time initially, a good interview is more likely to yield the information necessary to formulate a treatment plan.

By the time a child is referred for the assessment or treatment of a pain problem, the family has probably tried and failed to help the child effectively manage the pain. This means that they are almost certain to have strong feelings about the situation. In many medical settings, families perceive the referral to a mental health specialist as an implicit message that their child's pain is "all in her head." If so, they are likely to be angry and defensive, determined to convince you that their child's pain is "real." This reaction is very likely if the pain referral is made at the end of a lengthy medical work-up that yielded no clear medical etiology for the child's pain. The implied message to the parents in such situations is, "The doctors couldn't find anything medically wrong, so they gave up and referred the child to a shrink." Convinced that the doctors simply were not thorough enough, many parents will seek a second, third, or fourth medical opinion until they are certain that their child has been given serious consideration. The clinician can save hours of frustrating and fruitless interviews with defensive and angry parents by ascertaining their attitudes regarding mental health involvement up front.

One can also counter some of these negative family attitudes in the initial session by offering an unsolicited explanation of the role of the pain management specialist. For example, I find the following explanation is palatable to most parents, regardless of the underlying medical factors affecting their child's pain:

> I am a clinical psychologist. I am also a pain specialist. Dr. _____
> asked me to see Johnny to see if any psychological pain management
> strategies might be useful in helping him cope with his pain. What I'd
> like to do today is begin to get as complete a picture as possible of what
> his pain is like for him and what it is like for you and your family. This
> is the first step in developing a pain management program that is spe-
> cifically designed to meet Johnny's individual needs.

This sort of an explanation bypasses some of the parents' resistance because it does not require them at this point to buy into any psychological causes of their child's pain problem.

Refining the Operational Definition of the Child's Pain Problem

The parents can be a valuable source of information regarding the child's pain problem. In the case of young children, the parents will be able to observe and describe many aspects of the child's pain behaviors that the child would be unaware of or unable to articulate. In older children and adolescents, there should be some congruence between parent and child reports, although parents of older children and adolescents are likely to have less firsthand information regarding the child's pain experience, since parents do not monitor the child's behavior as closely at this age.

In general, it is best to ask parents to provide specific, behavioral information, rather than generalizations. There are two reason for this recommendation: First, much of the important information that guides the development of an effective, individualized pain management program is gleaned from the assembly and integration of small pieces of information until a pattern is discovered that helps clarify the child's pain problem. Important details and corresponding precision are lost when people are asked to generalize. Furthermore, retrospective recall is never as accurate as immediate recall. Therefore, it is much more useful to ask specific questions, such as, "What did you do when Susie started to cry when she tried to get out of bed today?" rather than, "What do you usually do when Susie cries when she's in pain?"

Another common error during this assessment phase is asking parents to make inferences regarding the possible causes of certain pain behaviors. Consider, for example, the seemingly innocent question: "Does she seem to complain of pain to get attention?" Although this is certainly an important *hypothesis* to entertain, and one we will address later, asking the parents to make this assessment is quite problematic. First of all, if they had had this particular psychological conceptualization of the child's pain, they probably already would have handled the child's pain problem. Second, most people are poor objective observers of themselves and their families. Therefore, most parents do *not* think their child's pain is due to psychological factors. Furthermore, asking them to take a stand and say, "No, I don't think she does it for attention," sets the stage for confrontation and possible failure in the future, if the assessment does indeed reveal that adult attention might be reinforcing the child's pain behaviors. It is much more useful to ask parents for more objective information, such as descriptions of the child's behavior and descriptions of the behaviors of others. It is the clinician's responsibility (and expertise) to collect the data, interpret the patterns of interactions, and ultimately integrate the data to formulate the treatment plan.

Finally, the question itself, "Does she seem to complain of pain to get attention?" is not really appropriate. Children do not typically volitionally induce or fake pain in order to get attention. When attention is involved, it is usually a much more subtle process of inadvertent social reinforcement. This is very different from the typical lay understanding of "doing something for attention." Therefore, we recommend never insinuating that the child is demonstrating pain "for attention."

The parents can provide additional information regarding the same basic questions addressed with the child:

1 | When does the child have pain? Under what conditions or in what settings?
2 | What is the quality, frequency, intensity, and severity of the child's pain?
3 | What are the behavioral, biological, and social consequences of the child's pain?

The clinician should start with the current pain episode and try to get as much information as possible about this event, then work back in time.

The Setting

When did her pain start? What was she doing? Where was she? Who else was with her? How had she been feeling physically immediately prior to the onset of pain? How had she been feeling emotionally immediately prior to the onset of pain?

The Pain Response

How did you know she was in pain? What did she do? What did she say? Tell me what happened the last time she was in pain. Describe anything you can think of. Try to assess the duration of any pain behaviors (e.g., how long did she cry?), the frequency of any pain behaviors (e.g., how many times did she scream?), and the intensity or severity of the behaviors (e.g., could people outside the room hear her crying? Could you calm her down once she started crying? How long did it take?)

Once a clear picture of this particular pain episode emerges, one can ask the parent to describe the pain episode that preceded this one. After three or four such explicit descriptions, the clinician should have a fairly good sense of what the child is like when in pain as well as a rough idea of the current frequency of pain episodes. At this point it is appropriate to ask if the events the parent has just described are typical of the child's pain experiences. If not typical, the clinician should ask for a description of the most recent typical example and try to obtain a detailed chronology of this pain episode.

One should also ask for recent examples of pain behaviors in other settings. Common settings where one might expect pain behaviors to differ include hospital versus home, home versus school, weekend versus school day, morning versus evening, awake versus asleep, in bed versus out of bed, prone versus sitting or walking, and in the presence of mother, father, other adults, or peers. These distinctions may help clarify the nature of the pain problem and may provide clues to more effective management. If the pain involves medical procedures, the child's past history with any medical procedures, even mildly uncomfortable ones should be assessed. This will provide information regarding the duration and extent of the pain problem as well as the severity of the pain.

Consequences

What happens when the child is in pain? What does the child do next? How do others in the environment respond? Again, the clinician should not ask the parents to assess whether they pay attention to the child's pain or somehow reinforce it, but should simply ask for a chronological report of what was said and done. The clinician can then examine this information to refine hypotheses regarding the environmental consequences of the child's pain.

For example, does the child fall asleep after the backrub? Does the parent distract her with conversation? Is the child's horrible pain miraculously cured by the application of a cartoon character bandage? The timing and the sequence of events may also shed light on the underlying contingencies.

THE MEDICAL CONTEXT IN WHICH THE PAIN PROBLEM OCCURS

It is also important to understand the general medical context in which the child's pain occurs before proceeding with a more detailed pain assessment. For example, if this is the first significant pain experience in a young child, it may be much more frightening and have different emotional consequences for the family than if the pain is occurring in a child who has had juvenile rheumatoid arthritis for ten years. Similarly, postsurgical pain is likely to have different meaning and different emotional ramifications than pain of unknown origin or pain associated with an end-stage terminal illness.

The following are important questions to consider in clarifying the medical context of the pain problem.

1 | Does the child have an underlying medical condition? What is it? When was it diagnosed? What is the parents' understanding of the seriousness of the illness? What are their primary concerns regarding the illness?
2 | Is pain the primary problem for this child? Or is it a secondary problem associated with the underlying illness?
3 | When did the child first develop pain? What happened? Was the pain successfully managed?

Health care providers can help clarify the medical and physical context of the child's pain problem. By knowing something about the child's illness and medical treatment to date, the clinician can be better prepared to generate and test hypotheses about the child's pain. At the very minimum, the clinician should know the child's diagnosis and current medical status. If the child is receiving any medical treatment for the pain, the details of current therapies (e.g., how often is physical therapy recommended?) and the dose and schedules of any pain medications should be obtained. Dose and scheduling of any other medications, including over-the-counter preparations, also should be recorded. As one comes to know the child and family, there will be many more medical questions that may need to be addressed; however, these often can be deferred until a later time. It is imperative, however, that the clinician know what the physician's impression of the child's pain is and what the physician's impressions of the family's understanding of the child's pain is. This information may reveal misunderstandings or discrepancies between the family's and the medical staff's impressions. This is particularly important in cases where the family believes the child's pain signifies an extremely serious underlying pathology.

THE SOCIAL CONTEXT

The broader social environment of the child—the school, the neighborhood, and the community—also is an important contextual variable to consider. As is true in all aspects of clinical practice with children, environmental factors can have a significant impact on the consequences of pain, the meaning of the child's pain, ongoing stressors, available resources, and social supports. Cultural factors that may influence the expression of pain and attitudes toward pain management also should be considered.

Generating Hypotheses Regarding Physical Contributors to the Child's Pain

The next step in the pain conceptualization process involves generating as many hypotheses as possible to account for the child's pain. The purpose of distinguishing the hypothesis generation process from the data collection and treatment planning processes is to force the clinician to think creatively. The hypothesis generation process involves brainstorming, in which any and all ideas are considered fair game and are not censored at the beginning. This hypothesis generation process helps prevent therapist bias. Expectations and prejudices, as well as experience and habit, can lead the clinician to pursue only a restricted range of hypotheses without ever realizing it. It is extremely easy to design an evaluation that will only obtain data that serve to confirm one's biased hypotheses and will not elicit data that might be disconfirmatory. Therefore, the hypotheses generated at the preliminary stage of case conceptualization should be uncensored and exhaustive. All possibilities should be considered.

Generating multiple hypotheses becomes easier with experience, as the clinician becomes more sensitive to the subtle ways in which pain problems can develop and be maintained. This volume is designed to help guide the process by highlighting the general categories of hypotheses that should be considered. But, to be optimally effective, conceptualizations should be unique to the child, and thus at a level of detail far beyond the scope of any one book. The chapters that follow outline the important content areas for which hypotheses should be generated. An overview of all of the primary hypotheses that will be discussed in this text were presented in table form in Chapter 2 (Figure 2.2). Hypotheses also are summarized at the end of the chapters that follow and in the worksheet in Appendix A.

GENERATING HYPOTHESES REGARDING THE CHILD'S PHYSICAL PAIN

A number of physical factors should be considered as possible contributors to or exacerbators of a child's pain.

Is the Child Receiving Less than Optimal Pain Medication?

Unfortunately, the answer to this question often is, "yes." In current medical practice, it is rare that children are not offered any analgesia. However, it is common to find practitioners who are not aware of all of the options available to minimize pain in children or who are not comfortable prescribing medications for children (Bush, Holmbeck, & Cockrelli, 1989; Schechter, Allen & Hanson, 1986). In such instances, the full range of medications may not have been offered to the child, or the medications may not have been prescribed in the most effective manner.

Are Medications that Are Likely to Help the Child's Pain Not Being Used?

A good example of an often underutilized pain management agent is EMLA® (Eutetic Mixture of Local Anesthetics) cream. This is a relatively newly developed topical anesthetic, which can be used to numb the skin prior to starting an IV or giving a shot. It is routinely used in pediatric cancer settings, where children must undergo hundreds of venipunctures and intramuscular injections that can be painful and upsetting. However, with EMLA®, many children do not even feel the needle going into the skin. Such appropriate analgesia can make a tremendous difference in whether or not the child comes to fear the medical situation. However, in settings where invasive procedures are not common and in settings where few children are treated, staff may be unfamiliar with EMLA® and may not have it on hand.

Are Pain Medications Being Administered Inappropriately or in a Less than Ideal Manner?

Inappropriate Dose

This problem often becomes evident when the child initially appeared to benefit from the medication but no longer seems to experience the same level of relief. Sometimes, the cause for this is simple—the child has grown and the dose needs to be adjusted. The amount of medication needed to achieve the desired analgesia depends on the child's weight. A growth spurt can render a previously effective dose ineffective.

It is also possible that the physician prescribed a conservative dose of a medication. A higher dose of the same agent may be safe and more effective.

If medications have been used continuously for some time, *tolerance* can develop. This means that the body becomes accustomed to the medication and the same dose of the medication no longer causes the same level of effect. A higher dose will be needed to achieve the same level of pain relief. Anyone can experience tolerance if the same medication is used for an extended period of time.

Inappropriate Timing

Even if the appropriate medical agent is being used, it may not be administered in an appropriate or optimal manner. EMLA® cream, for example, must be applied approximately 1 hour before a painful needle stick in order to be effective. Sometimes, a knowledgeable but impatient health care professional or parent is too rushed to wait 60 minutes in order to prevent pain.

Inappropriate Scheduling

One of the worst (and most common) errors made in pain prescriptions is scheduling the medication on a p.r.n. (*pro re nata*, or "as needed") basis. Although intuitively one might think pain medications should only be taken when absolutely necessary, this actually is the worst way to provide pain relief. Pain medications are most effective with milder pain. The more severe the pain, the more medication required to alleviate it. If pain becomes too severe, it may not be possible to relieve it. Therefore, most pain management specialists recommend taking pain medication *before* the pain becomes severe or unbearable (Schechter, 1989).

In his now classic article on the undertreatment of pain in children, Schechter (1989) summarized several additional serious problems that p.r.n. schedules can cause. First, when pain medications are prescribed p.r.n. someone (usually the nurse) must make the judgment call that they are, indeed, needed. This often puts an undue burden on nurses, who may fear criticism for over-using medications. It also places a demand on the child to "prove" that he/she really needs the medication. P.r.n. schedules also feed into misinformed beliefs (e.g., "children don't experience pain," "pain is good for you; it builds character," or "if you tough it out it and go without medication, it will make you stronger"), which may lead adults to refuse or delay giving medications to children. In addition, the child may feel embarrassed when asking for the pain medication, or may not be able to communicate his/her needs clearly.

Conflicts among parents, medical staff, and children over whether or not the child truly needs the medication may then arise. Under these circumstances, it is very common for parents to encourage children to try to wait just a little longer before taking their medications. However, this suggestion will backfire if the child's pain escalates in the interim. To illustrate, an 8-year-old boy once told the author that he tried to wake himself up around 2:00 A.M. every night, because if he were asleep "his nurse would think he didn't need any pain medication" and would not give it to him. If this happened, he explained, by morning his pain would be unbearable and would be unlikely to diminish quickly in response to the medication.

Finally, a p.r.n. schedule may actually encourage pain behaviors. In effect, it gives children the message that they must show a lot of pain behaviors in order to receive pain medication.

Around-the-clock scheduling is a much more effective way of providing pain medication and avoids the pitfalls mentioned above. This scheduling system provides the medication at regularly scheduled intervals (e.g., every 4, 6, 8 hours), with the goal of preventing pain (McGrath, 1990). This predictable schedule should allow the child to relax and feel assured that the medications will be administered on a regular basis. It also does not require the child to act "sick" in order to get the medications.

Breakthrough Pain

Pain that returns before the next scheduled dose of around-the-clock medication is administered is called *breakthrough* pain. This can create almost as stressful a situation for the child as the p.r.n. medication schedule. For example, one patient knew her pain medication would only last four hours, yet her doses were scheduled at 6-hour intervals. The last 2 hours of each interval dragged by as she counted the minutes she had to wait before obtaining relief. During this waiting period, her anxiety also mounted, as she worried about the possibility that her medicine might not be ready when the time period was up. She would repeatedly ask her nurse whether it was time for her medication and ask for reassurance that she would bring it promptly.

Administration Problems

Although the consequences of missing a dose of medication can be very significant, many children still encounter problems adhering to their pain medication regimen. Adherence is likely to be most difficult for the medications that serve more prophylactic functions, since the negative consequences of missing a dose and/or the positive impact on the underlying disease might be delayed (Meichenbaum & Turk, 1987). For example, a Juvenile Rheumatoid Arthritis (JRA) patient frequently forgot to take his regularly scheduled anti-inflammatory medications. He typically only remembered to take the medications several hours later in the day when his joints started to hurt.

Medications may also be administered incorrectly because of misunder-stood instructions or simple errors in measurement. For example, the common household tablespoon is a notoriously unreliable measurement device, varying from 2.5 to 9 mL in volume in some studies (Mattar, Markello, & Yaffe, 1975). Children may not receive the correct dose of inaccurately measured medication. Screaming, spitting, and vomiting children also do not ingest the full amount of their prescribed medication.

In hospitals, one may be surprised to discover that an overworked nursing staff or pharmacy is delivering the child's pain medication late, resulting in break-through pain. At home, family schedules may make the prescribed medication schedule extremely difficult to follow, or they may find it difficult to keep track of the exact times the medications were given, resulting in delays and breakthrough pain.

Misconceptions and Fears

Children may fail to obtain all scheduled medications because of adherence difficulties mentioned previously, or there may be underlying misconceptions that make the child reluctant to use the medication or the parents reluctant to encourage the child to use it. Concerns about addiction are among the most common. Few parents (and too few physicians) understand the difference between *tolerance* and *addiction*. Drug *tolerance* means that, over time, the child needs increasing amounts of the medication in order to obtain the same effect. This is a physical re-action one may see in someone who uses pain medication over an extended period of time. Physical dependence is another potential consequence of prolonged use of a drug. The body comes to require the drug in order to function; physical with-drawal symptoms will occur if the drug is withdrawn. Tolerance and withdrawal symptoms are common in children who have taken narcotic pain agents for over 2 weeks and then stop taking them (McGrath, 1990).

However, the presence of tolerance or physical dependence does not consti-tute addiction. According to the *DSM-IV*, in *addiction* (or "substance dependence," which is the more current official term), the individual uses the medication for rea-sons other than pain management and taking the medication causes personal, so-cial, or occupational impairment. In addition, feelings of craving and difficulty controlling the use of the substance are common. In pain situations, appropriate medication actually improves functioning, rather than impairing it (Sees & Clark, 1993). Indeed, it is extremely rare for someone who uses pain medication for acute pain to become addicted (Schechter, 1989; McGrath, 1990).

Other beliefs that may interfere with taking medication include religious or philosophical attitudes. Alcoholics Anonymous (AA), for example, encourages participants to avoid all chemicals, especially any drugs or alcohol. Alternatively, family members may believe that "giving in" to pain and needing a medication is a sign of weakness. As a result, they may encourage the child to delay or forgo taking pain medications (Schechter, 1989).

Finally, pain medications may have side effects that are unpleasant or even frightening for children. Pain medications can cause nausea and diarrhea. The "out of it" sensation caused by some narcotics can be very unpleasant. Some of the agents that are used for pain management during invasive procedures can cause children to hallucinate or act very strangely. This can be frightening for the child and very upsetting for parents, especially if they are not prepared for the possibility. After such a harrowing experience, they may opt to discontinue the medication.

Are the Medications Unavailable?

Medications are of no use, no matter how appropriately and sensitively prescribed, if they are not available when the child needs them. Parents may not be able to afford the medication their child needs, but may be too embarrassed to admit it. The family may not have thought to bring an extra set of medications to the school for dispensing during the day. In some cases, someone other than the child may be using the child's pain medication.

Are Other Physical Factors Exacerbating the Child's Pain?

Protective Posturing

When pain is present or expected, a natural tendency is to try to avoid the pain. For example, a child may try not to move the painful body part in order to "protect" it from hurting, or may tighten her muscles in anticipation of a shot or a searing pain. This protective posturing can have detrimental effects. Muscle tension exacerbates pain in most invasive procedures. An intramuscular injection into a tense muscle hurts much more than the same injection into a flaccid muscle. Muscle tension goes hand in hand with vasoconstriction, which makes IV access much more difficult.

In more chronic pain situations, holding part of the body in an unnatural position to keep from experiencing pain may actually cause new pains to develop in the muscles straining to maintain the protective posture. Immobility is a particularly dangerous protective maneuver. Substantial muscle loss and weakness can occur after relatively short periods of immobility, resulting in new medical problems and new sources of discomfort. A vicious cycle can easily develop. The more the child remains in bed to avoid pain, the poorer the child's strength and stamina become. Thus movement is more likely to be uncomfortable, resulting in even greater efforts on the child's part to avoid moving.

Fatigue

Unremitting pain is both physically and emotionally exhausting. If the child cannot sleep because of pain, his or her ability to tolerate pain the next day is likely to be compromised. Sleep deprivation due to other factors, such as an uncomfortable bed or noisy environment, also should be considered.

Environmental Variables

Simple physical factors, such as sleeping on the couch or a very soft mattress, or working at a computer with poor back support, carrying 20 pounds of books from class to class, or having to climb several flights of stairs, may exacerbate the pain problem.

Scheduling of Activities

The way in which physical activities are scheduled also can exacerbate pain. Just as it is important not to wait until pain is unbearable before taking medication, it is important to schedule physical activities in manageable doses before pain becomes severe. Rest periods are crucial to allow the child to monitor physical sensations and determine if an activity should be terminated. In addition, many physical activities can be tolerated with less pain if appropriate physical therapy "comfort measures" are used in preparation for or in conjunction with the activity. For example, stretching and other warm-up exercises can prevent muscle soreness. A warm bath can do wonders for the morning stiffness of arthritis, making it much easier to get dressed for school.

Other Medications

Some drugs may indirectly affect the child's pain tolerance. For example, any medications that make the child more emotional, such as steroids, are likely to hamper the child's ability to tolerate pain.

Table 3.1 summarizes the primary hypotheses regarding physical contributors to children's pain presented in this chapter. For the therapist's convenience, these hypotheses also are presented in the Generating Hypotheses/Evaluation Planning Worksheet in Appendix A.

Table 3.1. Summary of Potential Hypotheses Regarding Physical Contributors to the Child's Pain

1. Is the child receiving less than optimal pain medication?
   - Are available methods not being used?
2. Are appropriate medications being administered inappropriately?
   - Is the current dose inappropriate?
   - Are medications being administered at inappropriate times?
   - Are the medications scheduled inappropriately?
     Are medications prescribed p.r.n.?
     Is the child experiencing breakthrough pain?
   - Is the child or family or staff having problems with adherence?
     Are doses late or fogotten?
     Is the medication measured inaccurately?
   - Are beliefs, concerns or misconceptions interfering with medication administration?
3. Are the pain medications unavailable?
   - Are finances preventing purchase of the medications?
   - Is someone else using the medication?
4. Are other physical factors exacerbating the child's pain?
   - Is protective posturing or muscle tension causing additional discomfort or interfering with movement?
   - Is fatigue interfering with pain coping efforts?
   - Are environmental factors exacerbating pain?
   - Is the child over-exerting, failing to use appropriate rest periods, or otherwise not following PT recommendations?
   - Are other medications or other physical problems affecting his/her emotional, cognitive, or behavioral functioning?

Generating Hypotheses Regarding Cognitive and Emotional Contributors to the Child's Pain

As outlined in Melzack and Wall's gate control theory (Melzack, 1993; Melzack & Wall, 1965), how a person thinks about pain can have a tremendous impact on how the individual experiences pain. This applies to everyone, not just individuals thought to have psychosomatic pain. Indeed, the entire notion of "psychosomatic" pain is obsolete. Scientists now know that psychological factors can affect almost all aspects of physiological functioning, from the level of heart rate down to basic T-cell immunological functioning (Oltmanns & Emery, 1998). Therefore, one must assume that, for every individual, psychological (cognitive and emotional) factors contribute in some way to the experience of pain. The important goal of the assessment process, therefore, is not to determine *if* psychological factors are playing a role for this individual, but rather to determine *how* psychological factors function for this particular individual. As part of this process, one can generate specific hypotheses regarding cognitive and emotional factors that might be contributing to or exacerbating the child's pain problem. The possible hypotheses described in this chapter are not exhaustive. They are intended to suggest areas of inquiry that may be important in understanding a child's pain experience.

IS THE CHILD'S ATTENTION FOCUSED ON THE PAIN?

As described earlier, gate control theory argues that, in order to experience pain, the child must cognitively process the pain stimuli. In other words, some attention must be directed toward the pain sensations in order to open the gate. If the child is focusing his/her attention almost exclusively on the pain stimuli, the experience of pain is likely to be the most extreme.

Even when efforts are made to help the child redirect attention away from the pain, careful assessment may reveal that these efforts are not effective. Such well-intended efforts often fail because they are developmentally inappropriate. A common example of developmentally inappropriate attention diversion is telling a child to use an uninteresting adult pain management technique, such as focusing on a spot on the wall. Another developmental error in attention diversion is expecting the child to use distraction to manage pain without any adult assistance. This requires a level of autonomy in affect regulation of which many pre-adolescent children are incapable. There are several studies in the literature documenting that children are less likely to use pain management coping strategies when adults do not prompt them to use them, even if these strategies had been working very effectively (e.g., Dahlquist, Gil, Armstrong, DeLawyer, Greene, & Wuori, 1986; Elliott & Olson, 1983). This phenomenon most likely reflects the fact that children, especially young children, need adults to help them regulate their affect (Kopp, 1982).

Attentional factors also can play a role in recurrent pain syndromes. Zeltzer (1995) argues that "some children are more aware of visceral sensations and interpret these sensations as 'pain'" (p. 280). For example, most children fleetingly notice body sensations associated with digestion but are not bothered by them. Children with recurrent abdominal pain, however, may interpret the same feelings of fullness or intestinal motility as "pain." Furthermore, they may focus their attention on these pain sensations and subsequently develop maladaptive pain behaviors (Zeltzer, 1995).

IS ANXIETY OR STRESS EXACERBATING THE CHILD'S PAIN?

The specific emotional states of children can be very difficult to determine. Because children lack the linguistic abilities to describe fine distinctions in their emotions, clinicians must infer their emotional state from their behavior. Often, anxiety, fear, and pain become intertwined in the child's distress behaviors and are indistinguishable to the adult observer. Sometimes, one can see the confounding effects, such as when a child says "ouch" before her mother touches the hairbrush to her tangled ponytail. Other times, one cannot tell if the child is crying from fear, pain, or both. At the very least, it is important to consider the possibility that the child is anxious or frightened, since these emotions will certainly exacerbate the pain experience.

Are Aspects of the Child's Environment Frightening?

Is the child in an unfamiliar environment? Have people failed to explain what is happening and what the child can expect? Are important adults in the child's life crying or frightened or absent? Any of these factors can create an atmosphere of fear that could exacerbate any pain the child experiences.

Are Clear Signals for the Onset and Termination of Painful Stimuli Lacking?

Predictability is crucial in helping one adapt to a painful stimulus. In one study, simply turning on a light before a painful medical experience helped a young girl tolerate multiple intensive care unit medical procedures without excessive fear or pain (Derrickson, Neef, & Cataldo, 1993). Yet, many parents and health care providers erroneously fear that telling a child when something will hurt will make things worse. Consequently, they often try to "sneak" the painful event in without alerting the child, for example, giving children chemotherapy injections at home while they are sleeping. Unfortunately, this strategy usually backfires, and the child experiences a sense of uncertainty and fear that the pain could come at any time.

Does the Pain Increase under Stressful Conditions?

Since negative emotions such as anxiety, frustration, depression, and anger may precipitate or exacerbate pain (Martin, Milech, & Nathan, 1993; O'Brien & Haynes, 1995), the child's pain is likely to be greatest in stressful situations. For children, this pattern is typically evident in school. It is very common for children's pain to be worse on school days or worse at a particular time of day that corresponds with a difficult class or difficult social situation in the school environment (such as lunchtime).

Allen and Matthews (1998) argue that "children with recurrent abdominal pain have different predispositions or thresholds of responsiveness to environmental stress that activate a poorly regulated nervous system" (p. 264). It is the interaction between the organism's vulnerability and the environmental stress that results in pain episodes. Thus, migraine patients tend to demonstrate neurovascular reactivity to stress, while recurrent abdominal patients respond with greater gastrointestinal reactivity (Allen & Matthews, 1998). If a stress relationship is evident, the therapist may need to eliminate sources of stress or help the child develop better ways to manage his/her physiological reactions to the stress.

DOES THE CHILD ENGAGE IN SELF-DEFEATING THINKING ABOUT THE PAIN?

A common pitfall for both adults and children, catastrophic or negative thinking can exacerbate a pain situation. For example, a child who says to himself, "I can't stand this!" or "I'll never get any sleep!" is not likely to use any pain management strategies. Adults may also communicate negative messages, such as "Only babies cry," which can lead the child to see himself as incapable of handling the pain. Regardless of whether these hopeless, helpless feelings are specific to the challenge of the pain situation or are more pervasive, they are likely to interfere with persistent efforts to manage pain. For example, children with sickle cell disease who reported negative thinking when they had pain (e.g., catastrophizing, fear self-statements, and anger self-statements) were less active, experienced greater psychological distress, and required more health care services during pain episodes than children who used more active coping strategies (Gil, Williams, Thompson, & Kinney, 1991; Gil, Thompson, Keith, Tota-Faucette, Noll, & Kinney, 1993).

DOES THE PAIN HAVE SIGNIFICANT EMOTIONAL MEANING FOR THE CHILD?

Children may have convoluted and unexpected beliefs about their illness, which may add a significant emotional valence to the pain situation. For example, children often fear that they are going to need surgery or some other serious medical intervention because of their pain, and are therefore quite frightened. If the child fears he or she is dying, the pain takes on a different emotional significance than if the pain is associated with a sports injury. Even if the adults in the child's life are not distressed by the pain, the child may have fears or misconceptions that need to be addressed.

Conversely, younger children may not be cognitively able to understand or speculate about the nature of their illness. However, they can be extremely sensitive to the emotions communicated by their caregivers. If the parent is frightened by the child's pain, the child is likely to sense this. Caregiver attitudes often are communicated indirectly by efforts to help the child deal with the pain. For example, worried parents who attempt to offer comfort and reassurance may actually communicate their own anxiety as their voices get louder and more strained as they almost desperately repeat, "It's OK, it's OK, it's OK!" (Gelfand, Dahlquist, & Hass, 1998). Consequently, one needs to consider the emotional meaning of the child's pain for the child as well as for the caregiver. The caregiver may well feel inadequate and anxious if he or she is unable to help the child cope with the pain.

IS THE CAREGIVER'S EMOTIONAL OR COGNITIVE STATUS INTERFERING WITH HIS/HER ABILITY TO HELP THE CHILD MANAGE THE PAIN?

This is a related factor that is often overlooked in pain assessment. It will do little good to develop an elegant pain management program requiring intensive parent

Table 4.1. Summary of Potential Hypotheses Regarding Cognitive and Emotional Contributors to the Child's Pain

1. Is the child's attention focused on the pain?
   - Are potential sources of distraction not being utilized in a developmentally appropriate manner?
2. Is anxiety exacerbating the child's pain?
   - Are aspects of the child's environment frightening?
   - Are clear signals for the onset and termination of painful stimuli lacking?
3. Does the child engage in self-defeating thinking about the pain?
4. Does the pain have significant emotional meaning for the child?
5. Is the caregiver's emotional or cognitive status interfering with his/her ability to assist the child in managing the pain?

participation if the parent is so depressed by an impending divorce, or so upset about the child's illness that he or she cannot concentrate on the child's situation.

A summary of the primary hypotheses regarding cognitive and emotional contributors to pain in children is presented in Table 4.1. The hypotheses also are included in the Hypothesis Generation/Testing Worksheet in Appendix A.

Generating Hypotheses Regarding Behavioral Contributors to the Child's Pain

The main hypotheses proposed in this chapter are guided by fundamental principles of learning. These principles can be summed up in five main questions:

1	To what degree is the problem behavior (i.e., pain behavior) positively reinforced?
2	To what degree is the problem behavior negatively reinforced?
3	Is the desired behavior (i.e., pain management behaviors, or maintaining adaptive functioning) somehow punished?
4	Is there inadequate reinforcement for the desired behavior?
5	Does the child lack the skills necessary for the desired adaptive behavior?

Each of these questions should be addressed from both the standpoint of the child, and from the more often neglected standpoint of the child's family. We will consider the child first.

PAIN BEHAVIOR IN CHILDREN

Before examining specific learning-based hypotheses to account for the child's pain, we must first specify what is considered actual pain behavior. In general, anything that indicates pain should be considered pain behavior. Crying and complaining that something hurts are pain behaviors as are vocalizations of discomfort, such as whimpering, groaning, and moaning. Protective posturing, holding a limb so it doesn't move, flinching, grimacing, holding one's breath, rubbing a muscle, pulling on an ear, tensing, or limping can all be nonverbal signs of pain.

Any combination of pain behaviors can be maintained by environmental consequences.

TO WHAT DEGREE IS THE CHILD'S PAIN BEHAVIOR POSITIVELY REINFORCED?

In other words, does the child's pain behavior result in pleasant or otherwise desired events that increase the likelihood of the pain behaviors occurring again? Some degree of positive reinforcement of pain behavior is almost inevitable, given the tendency of adults to respond in a protective manner to a child in pain. Pain behaviors, at the minimum, are noticed by adults, and attention, in and of itself, can be an extremely powerful reinforcer. The attention may take the form of comments or questions about pain ("Does your tummy hurt today?"), or time with the parent at home to recuperate. More subtle reinforcers include coming to the child's side when he/she winces in pain, or hovering lest the child need something. Cards, gifts, and visits from friends and family can make a painful event seem almost festive. Additional reinforcers include hugs and kisses, holding and rocking, stroking, and otherwise physically and verbally comforting the child.

For an event to serve as a positive reinforcer, it is not necessary for the level of reinforcement to be deficient initially. Certainly, there are cases where this is true, such as the busy parent who only spends time with the child when sick or en route to the doctor. But, more often, the positive reinforcement occurs in the context of responsive parenting and a nurturing environment, where the timing of parental attention inadvertently becomes tied to the child's pain complaints.

In identifying reinforcers in the child's environment it is important to take into account the current schedule of reinforcement. Does the parent respond the same way every time the child complains of pain, or is the attention intermittent, and thus more resistant to extinction?

TO WHAT DEGREE IS THE CHILD'S PAIN BEHAVIOR NEGATIVELY REINFORCED?

Does the pain behavior enable the child to escape or avoid something unpleasant? Negative reinforcers can be more difficult to identify because the "unpleasant" aspect of the avoided situation may not be known. For example, one 10-year-old chronic abdominal pain patient was an excellent student with many friends at school. She said she liked her teacher and had always enjoyed going to school. Therefore, no one suspected any negative reinforcement of her pain complaints. However, she had been absent from school for several weeks while being evaluated at the hospital. As a result, she had fallen behind in her schoolwork. Always something of a perfectionist, she was horrified that she would not get straight A's and at the same time overwhelmed by the magnitude of the work she would face upon returning to school. Although there was a documented physical cause for her stomach pain, her pain complaints were, to some degree, also maintained by the fact that they enabled her to continue to stay home from school and avoid the stress of make-up work and the possibility of substandard grades.

Pain behaviors also may be strengthened by the simple fact that they sometimes diminish the intensity of the child's pain or allow the child to avoid experiencing pain. Staying in bed or refusing to move a painful arm or leg are good examples of behaviors that may temporarily enable the child to avoid pain. Children who have had gastroenteritis may develop heightened sensitivity to internal sensations they have come to associate with severe gastrointestinal pain. These children may show dramatic pain avoidance behaviors, such as bending over in apparent distress, whenever their stomach growls. The doubling over behavior may become strengthened by the apparent avoidance of abdominal pain.

During medical procedures, pain behaviors often are inadvertently reinforced by the fact that they delay the start of the procedure. The crying, protesting child may be yelled at, threatened, or even spanked, but in the meantime, the child is *not* receiving the shot. Thus, the avoidance or delay of the painful shot negatively reinforces the child's protest behaviors.

Clinicians also should consider the possibility that recurrent pain problems are maintained because they allow the child to escape the responsibility of managing his/her pain (Allen & Matthews, 1995). It can take considerable effort to manage pain. It is much easier to cry and lay in bed and let a parent bring the pain medications, give back rubs, and do the child's household chores.

IS ADAPTIVE BEHAVIOR INADEQUATELY REINFORCED OR ACTUALLY PUNISHED?

This may seem to be an odd question, but it is important to consider. If the child stops complaining of pain, will his/her life become more negative? Will all the cards and toys and visits stop? Will Mom go back to work and stop spending one-on-one time with him? Will his older brother revert to his old patterns of picking on him and taking his toys? Will he have to return to school, where he will be teased whenever he reads aloud?

Adaptive coping with pain can be punished even in subtle ways. For example, a child who remains in good spirits despite pain may not receive her pain medicaiton. In such cases, the child quickly learns to maintain pain behaviors to prevent the medication from being taken away.

Similarly, relaxation or distraction exercises may not be used if met with criticism or ridicule. One father once told us that our pain management program was "ridiculous and he wasn't going to bother having his child do such a foolish thing." There was no point in recommending such strategies for this child, as long as his parent continued to hold these beliefs. In another case with a pre-teen patient, the author spent several sessions teaching her relaxation strategies to use before and during chemotherapy injections. The girl was given a tape recorder and headphones, so she could listen to the relaxation tape in the clinic waiting room. However, the girl refused to comply with this pain management strategy because she was too embarrassed to wear the headphones in public, fearing that people would think she was a "geek." Thus, the patient thought she would be punished (i.e., via ridicule) if she complied with the pain management behavior.

DOES THE CHILD LACK THE SKILLS NECESSARY TO PERFORM THE ADPATIVE BEHAVIOR(S)?

Some children may not demonstrate adaptive behaviors because the contingencies support pain behaviors rather than more adaptive functioning. However, even if the contingencies supported adaptive behaviors, many children could not function more adaptively because they lack the necessary skills. No changes in contingencies will help the child who does not know how to behave appropriately. Therefore, it is crucial to identify and remediate skill deficits.

Although it is beyond the scope of this book to identify all possible areas of skill deficits that can affect adaptive functioning in children, the most common problems that are associated with pain behaviors will be highlighted.

Cognitive and Academic Deficits

Since the main "job" of children is to attend school, deficits that interfere with academic functioning often may influence pain problems. Deficits in general intelligence, study skills, academic knowledge, attention, memory, and specific learning disabilities, to name just a few examples, can hamper the child's ability to perform well in school. If regular school attendance is the desired goal for a child with chronic pain, it is essential to determine whether the child has the cognitive and academic skills necessary to succeed in the classroom. This hypothesis should be posed any time school attendance or performance is of concern, regardless of whether or not pain behaviors are problematic. Cognitive skills can also limit the degree to which the child is capable of anticipating problem situations and planning appropriate responses.

Social and Communication Skills Deficits

For many children with chronic pain conditions, pain behaviors actually serve a variety of communicative functions. In fact, the pain behaviors may become the primary way of expressing their emotional experiences. Consider the toddler, who reports a "tummy ache" on the first day of school. The "tummy ache" may reflect his/her understandable apprehension about the new preschool, expressed concretely due to unsophisticated abstract thinking abilities and language skills. The sensitive parent or teacher will sense the child's uncertainty and fears and provide reassurance in response to this indirect communication of emotion. The parent also may begin to teach verbal labeling of affect and verbal communication of emotions by saying, "I think your tummy is upset because you are nervous about your new school. Once you meet your teacher and get to know the new children, I bet you won't feel so scared and your tummy will probably start to feel better." However, if the child does not learn alternative ways to express emotions as he or she grows up, pain behaviors may continue to serve an important emotional communication function. Pain behaviors may remain the primary means for communicating emotions and obtaining support, and more adaptive skills for communication may not develop.

It is also possible that the parent or others in the child's environment have communication skills deficits. The parent may not be sensitive to emotional cues in the child or may not know how to respond to the child's more subtle communication of emotions. The more obvious, dramatic pain behaviors may be the only cues to which the parent knows how to respond.

ADULT RESPONSES TO THE CHILD'S PAIN

The way the adults involved with the child respond to the child's pain also can be conceptualized from a learning theory perspective, although the questions need to be reframed somewhat. If we consider the problematic adult behavior as reinforcement of child pain behaviors or failure to reinforce child coping behaviors, the hypotheses can be rephrased in the following manner:

1   To what degree is the adult's problematic behavior positively reinforced?
2   To what degree is the adult's problematic behavior negatively reinforced?
3   Is the appropriate adult behavior (i.e., appropriately reinforcing the child's adaptive functioning) somehow punished?
4   Is there inadequate reinforcement for appropriate adult behavior?

The interactions between parents and children are complex and reciprocal. In many cases, the child's behavior serves to reinforce the parent's behavior. External factors also play a role. Both factors need to be considered when generating hypotheses.

To What Degree Is the Adult's Problematic Behavior Positively Reinforced?

Does the parent receive support and attention from the medical staff? Does he/she get support and attention from friends and family while the child is ill? Do the special needs of the child give the parent a sense of importance or competence or special status? For example, the lonely, isolated parent of a child with an intractable pain problem was in daily contact with supportive staff and patients who sympathized with her situation. Even in periods of robust health, this woman looked for signs of pain in her child, often seeking multiple evaluations of minuscule complaints in order to meet her own emotional needs for companionship and attention.

On a more simplistic level, it feels good to comfort a child. To quell their tears or hold them close can meet many adults' needs to feel needed and important, not to mention loved.

To What Degree Is the Adult's Problematic Behavior Negatively Reinforced?

Family therapists have long recognized the function that pain problems can serve in a disturbed family system. A teenager unable to sleep alone because of her pain can very effectively enable her mother to avoid sexual relations with her husband and thereby avoid confronting the problems in their marriage. A child in pain may enable the parent to stay home from an unpleasant or stressful job.

In many cases, the termination of the child's noxious behavior negatively reinforces the parent's problematic behavior. The child stops complaining of pain or stops crying in response to the adult's ministrations, thereby negatively reinforcing the parent's behavior.

Is Appropriate Adult Behavior Inadequately Reinforced or Somehow Punished?

Unfortunately, parents can be punished for appropriately trying to help their child manage his/her pain or get on with his/her daily activities. Relatives and friends frequently criticize parents for being harsh and insensitive if they try to ignore pain behaviors, or send a child to school despite pain. If the parents have any uncertainty or ambivalence themselves, such criticism can sabotage any efforts to change the way they handle the child's pain. The child may also unwittingly punish the parents' efforts to ignore pain behaviors by crying harder and longer in an effort to get attention.

Table 5.1. Summary of Potential Hypotheses Regarding Behavioral Contributors to the Child's Pain

1. To what degree is the child's pain behavior positively reinforced?
2. To what degree is the child's pain behavior negatively reinforced?
3. Is adaptive behavior inadequately reinforced or punished?
4. Does the child lack the skills necessary to perform the adaptive behavior?
   - Cognitive/academic deficits?
   - Social/communication deficits?
5. To what degree is the adult's problematic behavior positively reinforced?
6. To what degree is the adult's problematic behavior negatively reinforced?
7. Is appropriate adult behavior inadequately reinforced or punished?

Table 5.1 summarizes the general behavioral hypotheses covered in this chapter. The Hypothesis Generation and Testing Worksheet in Appendix A also includes these behavioral hypotheses.

6

Developing an Evaluation Plan

After an exhaustive list of hypotheses to account for the child's pain has been generated, the next step in the evaluation process involves testing each hypothesis. The therapist collects data from the child, the family, the medical staff, and others in the child's environment, and then examines the accumulated evidence to determine the degree to which each hypothesis is supported or refuted. As this process unfolds, the therapist builds an array of supporting and refuting data until each hypothesis has been tested.

The information collected in this assessment phase is guided by the specific hypotheses that have been generated. Standard, generic assessments sometimes used in other clinical settings, such as a standard battery of IQ, personality, and academic measures, may be of little value in this problem-oriented evaluation process, because they will not address the specific, idiographic kinds of hypotheses that need to be tested to understand and treat the child's pain problem.

For each hypothesis, the therapist should have an idea of (1) the types of information that could be useful in testing the hypothesis and (2) the ways in which he/she might obtain such information. In other words, if this hypothesis were true, what behaviors would you expect from the child, from the parents, from others in the family? What information would suggest that this hypothesis is not true? How can you get this information? What would be the most efficient way to get this information? Once these questions have been answered, this component of the evaluation can be planned. The therapist should then move on to the next hypothesis.

Before any assessment sessions beyond the initial interview take place, a comprehensive evaluation plan should be developed based on the specific hypotheses generated for the case. The plan should include an outline of what information is needed, the various methods by which the information can be obtained, and a prioritization of the methods determined to be the most useful as well as the order in which the therapist plans to obtain the information. (See the Evaluation Planning Worksheet in Appendix A.)

Let us consider, for example, one of the hypotheses we proposed for a child presenting with severe distress during chemotherapy injections. *Are clear signals for the onset and termination of the painful stimulus lacking?* Information that would suggest that this hypothesis is true would be any indication that the injections were given in an unpredictable manner, thus leaving the child to wonder when she was going to feel pain. Evidence of a clear signal prior to the needle stick would suggest that the hypothesis is false. Possible sources of such information included an interview with the child, interview with the parent, interview with the nurse giving the shot, and direct observation of the injection. However, since the participants in the process may not be very attentive to the actual behaviors of the nurse immediately preceding the shot, direct observation of an injection probably would be the most useful way to test this hypothesis.

Although the process of determining exactly what data are needed to test each hypothesis may seem cumbersome, in actuality this process is extremely efficient. By planning up front exactly what one needs to learn about the child, the information obtained during each evaluation session can be maximized. A thorough plan will eliminate repeated calls to the physician or nurse and will ensure that any self-monitoring data obtained will be optimally useful. Such efficiency can be essential if the child's insurance company limits the number of evaluation sessions that will be reimbursed. Professionals also have an ethical responsibility not to waste the patient's time and money by conducting poorly planned and minimally informative evaluation sessions.

For the inexperienced clinician, the comprehensive evaluation plan provides a reassuring structure for the next few sessions. The information to be gleaned is clear, and the plan for obtaining this information also is clear. If the clinician is unsure of how to test a specific hypothesis, the areas where consultation is needed also are apparent from the assessment plan.

An additional benefit of this evaluation approach involves structuring the therapy process. The clinician should clearly communicate to the patient and family that treatment will not begin until the evaluation stage is completed. Following the evaluation, the therapist will then present the findings and the resulting conceptualization and treatment plan to the family (and medical personnel, if appropriate). If all parties agree with the plan, psychological treatment will then proceed. By structuring the therapy process in this manner, one avoids unrealistic expectations for improvement before actual treatment begins. Most psychologists probably have had patients complain that "therapy isn't helping at all," when actually they were still conducting the evaluation. Clarifying the evaluation process ahead of time helps avoid these misunderstandings. By proposing a specific treatment plan and explaining the underlying conceptualization before beginning treatment, the therapist also engages the family in a partnership of sorts.

Finally, by establishing the underlying conceptual framework for the proposed treatment first, one can determine if the family's views are too incompatible with the therapist's to allow them to accept the proposed treatment. Obviously, conceptualizations should be framed in ways to be optimally understood and accepted by family members. But, if serious misgivings will interfere with their cooperation, one should address this at the start, rather than discovering it as the reason behind noncompliance and frustration weeks into treatment.

Presenting the conceptualization may also actually begin the therapy process, if indeed there is evidence suggesting that ignorance or misinformation is contributing to the pain problem. The therapist may want to begin with corrective information (i.e., regarding the addictive potential of certain medications, or the role of stress in exacerbating pain) as part of the conceptual rationale.

In the chapters that follow, suggestions are offered for ways that one might test the hypotheses that are discussed in the preceding chapters. The types of information that can be helpful and some of the pros and cons of different methods of obtaining such information are provided. These guidelines are designed to provide the clinician unfamiliar with pain management with a starting point for generating a conceptualization that is unique to the individual child. However, these guidelines are not exhaustive. Although many of the same questions can be posed for similar types of pain problems, these guidelines should not be taken as a simple "cookbook." Once the clinician stops thinking creatively about the individual child, important data unique to the child will be lost. Thus, when following these guidelines and suggestions, they should be tailored to the specific needs of each patient. For example, is a chart on the refrigerator, or a checklist page in the day planner, or an index card inside the lunch box, or a phone call to the therapist's voice mail the best way to obtain self-reported pain intensity ratings from this particular child? The goal here should be to create the optimal assessment method for the specific hypotheses that have been generated for this particular child, rather than picking a generic measure.

Measuring the Child's Pain

In order to test any hypotheses about factors related to the child's pain, the clinician must have a good sense of when the child is in pain, and how the child's subjective pain experience as well as the child's observable pain behaviors vary, depending on different aspects of the situation. These variations will provide some of the most important evidence supporting or refuting hypotheses regarding the child's pain problem. Data regarding pain behaviors can be obtained from multiple sources, including the observations of adults in the environment and direct observation. However, by definition, information about subjective experiences can only be obtained from the child. Therefore, it is important to develop an assessment approach that measures the child's pain experience as accurately as possible.

Developmental factors are the most important determinants of how one should approach the ongoing measurement of the child's subjective pain.[*] This chapter describes possible ways to measure each of the dimensions of pain experience: location, frequency, duration, quality, and intensity. In general, however, we have had little success with routine use of any written pain assessment strategies (even very simple ones) in children under the age of 5. Their attention spans are too fleeting, and they are so easily distracted by other aspects of scribbling on paper that it is very difficult to obtain any consistent pain report in this format. Therefore, we recommend relying entirely on verbal report for children under the age of 5. However, older children may be able to provide additional information via written self-reports.

Regardless of the format of the self-report methodology, it is important to be sure that the child gives careful attention to the rating. These self-reports are not likely to be intrinsically interesting or important to most children. They are likely to rush through them and complete them carelessly. This doesn't mean that they do not care about improving their pain. It just means that they will need structure (and perhaps rewards) for careful completion of any records. Even adolescents will need some structure and incentives, especially if recordkeeping is ongoing and lasts for a long time.

[*] For a more extensive discussion of developmental issues in pain assessment in children, see Ross and Ross (1988), McGrath (1990), Thompson and Varni (1986), or Dahlquist (1990).

LOCATION OF PAIN

Even very young children can give a general indication of where they hurt by pointing. Sometimes one needs to listen carefully to understand what their limited vocabulary is trying to convey. For example, some creative 3-year-olds may say: "My neck hurts" (sore throat), "My ear is scratchy" (middle ear infection), "I hurt all over" (high fever).

It is simplest to ask the child to point to the part on their body that hurts. Until the child is cognitively able to picture an object from various perspectives other than his or her own, it will be very confusing to try to mark on a picture a sore area corresponding to a spot on his or her body. However, after about age 7, making an "X" or coloring a spot on a drawing of a body may be an additional useful way to keep track of body areas that hurt. Such a strategy may be particularly useful for illnesses such as juvenile rheumatoid arthritis, in which multiple joints in the body may be painful at different times. Obviously, if the child has pain in only one body part (e.g., a headache) or at an injection site, continuing to assess pain location will be of little utility.

The degree to which one can determine the quantitative aspects of the child's pain experience will depend on the level at which the child understands various numerical and time constructs. Although acquisition of these constructs varies considerably and depends on education and experience, some general guidelines can be suggested.

INTENSITY OF PAIN

Preschoolers typically understand the concept of relative size in a very simple form. They can identify which object is bigger than another or pick out the biggest item in an array. It becomes more difficult when they are asked to specify gradations of size. For example, the three-level ranking of "big, smaller, smallest" may not emerge until age 4. However, the metric used to measure the magnitude of emotional stimuli does not necessarily parallel that of the physical world. For preschoolers, virtually any hurt is a "big" hurt, especially when it is happening. If the hurt is accompanied by blood, it is almost guaranteed to be a "big" hurt. Arguing with a young child that the tiny, albeit bleeding, paper cut is not nearly as bad as the nasty gash he received last week when he fell down the stairs is of no use.

This limitation is important to keep in mind when evaluating the outcome of any intervention for pain in young children. It will be difficult to get a clear indication of pain intensity from children under the age of 5 or 6. For older children, variations of visual analog scales can be used on a repeated basis to monitor variations in perceived pain intensity.

For a 6-year old, one may consider the following phrasing:

How much did the shot hurt?
    no hurt _____ very big hurt
For older children, more abstract anchors can be used.
How much did the shot hurt?
    no pain _____ very severe pain
How much did the shot hurt?
    no pain _____ worst pain possible

We do not recommend using numerical ratings (i.e., "On a scale of 0 to 100, with 0 meaning no pain and 100 meaning the worst possible pain, how bad was your pain this morning?") until the child is very comfortable manipulating numbers of this magnitude in a variety of situations. Indicators of readiness include being able to use money, calculate change, and manipulate fractions easily. Children are not expected to have mastered these skills until the fifth or sixth grade.

Simplified rating scales, such as 4- or 5-point Likert scales, also have been used with some success in children over the age of 8 or 9. Descriptors typically accompany the Likert ratings. The child is asked to circle the number that fits the severity of his/her pain. Examples of such scales are presented in Figure 7.1.

FREQUENCY OF PAIN

In the development of the initial operational definition of the child's pain problem, the approximate frequency of the child's pain should have become evident. The way in which one measures ongoing pain frequency in the hypothesis testing

---

How bad is your headache?

0	1	2	3	4
No headache	Mild	Painful	Severe	Very severe

How bad is your headache?

0 = No headache
1 = Only aware of it if I pay attention to it
2 = Able to ignore it sometimes
3 = Can't ignore it but I can do most activities
4 = Difficult to concentrate, I can only do easy activities
5 = So severe, I can't do anything

Figure 7.1. Likert scales for pain intensity ratings. (Adapted from Richardson, McGrath, Cunningham, & Humphreys, 1983.)

phase should reflect the clinician's sense of the general frequency of the child's pain. Thus, there is no point in asking for hourly pain estimates if the child only has one or two headaches per week. However, estimates should be obtained as close to the time that the pain occurs as is possible, to maximize the accuracy of the child's recall.

For example, for pain that occurs approximately once a day, a calendar may be used to record pain-free days and days the child experiences pain. (See Figure 7.2.) More frequently occurring pain should be monitored more often. Again, the developmental level of the child will influence the format this takes. It may only be reasonable to ask younger children to provide ratings for few time periods, such as in the morning, after lunch, after dinner, and nighttime. Alternatively, one may choose to anchor the ratings to specific activities, such as getting dressed, boarding the bus, during first period, during lunch, after school, after dinner, getting in bed, etc. Adolescents may be able to provide hourly ratings (if the incentives are powerful enough) which combine frequency with other dimensions of the pain experience. (See Figure 7.3.)

DURATION OF PAIN

Estimates of duration are most useful if the child experiences discrete pain episodes. For example, headaches and morning stiffness are good examples of pain episodes that would be expected to vary in duration from day to day. If the child has a good sense of time, he or she may be able to estimate the duration of a pain episode at the end of the day. Otherwise, one can ask the child to record the time the pain started and the time it stopped. If time is too abstract a concept, the child may be able to give an approximation of duration by anchoring start and stop times with daily events. For example, did the pain start before breakfast? After he got to school? After lunch? Similarly, did the pain end before math class? After dinner? Sometime during the night?

QUALITY OF PAIN

Qualitative aspects of the child's pain are difficult to assess via diaries unless the child is an adolescent and has the vocabulary to make fine discriminations between sensory descriptions (e.g., searing versus dull and throbbing). We have found it more useful to rely on interviews to explore the sensory quality of the pain experience. At the minimum, one should attempt to understand the sensations the child experiences at the start of the evaluation and then any time the nature of the pain experience seems to change. This is especially important if there are multiple pain sites, since there may be different factors contributing to the different sites of pain. For example, a child complaining of migraine pain may subsequently de-

Date _____

Time	Setting	Activity	Location of pain	Intensity (0–100)	Duration (minutes)	What did you do to decrease the pain?	Effectiveness (0–100%)	Tension (1–10)

Figure 7.2. Daily pain diary.

Date_____

Time	Rate pain intensity in each area (0–100)									Setting	Activity	Mood	Tension (1–10)	Pain relief attempted
	Head	Neck	Chest	Back	Arms (R,L)	Hands (R,L)	Stomach	Legs (R,L)	Feet (R,L)					
8:00–9:00														
9:00–10:00														
10:00–11:00														
11:00–12:00														
12:00–1:00														
1:00–2:00														
2:00–3:00														
3:00–4:00														
4:00–5:00														
5:00–6:00														
6:00–7:00														
7:00–8:00														
8:00–9:00														
9:00–10:00														
10:00–11:00														
Night														

Figure 7.3. Hourly pain ratings.

velop backaches secondary to sleeping on the couch. Some children will be able to distinguish between the "throbbing" pain of a migraine and the "dull ache" of a poorly supported back. However, there is considerable variability in children's abilities to communicate qualitative distinctions in pain. In many cases, we find this aspect of pain is less reliable and less useful than pain intensity and frequency ratings.

PAIN-FREE PERIODS

After suffering with pain for any length of time, the periods of relief and relative comfort are often forgotten. However, as the sections that follow will illustrate, the pain-free periods may well provide important clues to causes or potential treatments for the pain problem. Therefore, it may be equally important to have the child identify periods, however brief they might be, when the pain remits or is absent. Formats similar to the ones provided above can be adapted to yield data regarding pain-free periods as well.

GOALS OF ASSESSMENT

The main objective of the hypothesis testing phase of the pain evaluation is to accumulate evidence that will either support or refute hypotheses regarding the child's pain. Therefore, one must be thorough and objective, so that possible unexpected findings are not precluded from consideration or overlooked. One of the best ways to ensure that this does not happen is to obtain information regarding *multiple examples* of pain experiences and to use *multiple sources* of information. Multiple examples prevent erroneous conclusions from being drawn from a single, unrepresentative event. Furthermore, patterns in behavior (such as intermittent reinforcement of pain behavior) are difficult to detect until several instances are observed. Multiple sources of information help minimize the possibility that the observer or reporter may have missed crucial information or misinterpreted certain events because of personal emotions or bias.

Obviously, behavioral patterns will not become apparent if the child's pain report does not vary, for example, if the child reports that his pain is a "10" on a 10-point scale all of the time, regardless of the situation. In such cases, the pain diary reveals more about the child's efforts to communicate his/her emotional distress than information about the child's pain in particular.

Whenever possible, the clinician should strive to get moment-by-moment accounts or directly observe the child, so that the data available are as objective as possible, rather than someone's interpretation of the events. Information regarding various individuals' *interpretations* of the situation can be reserved for the evaluation of hypotheses regarding the contributions of beliefs and attitudes to the child's pain problem.

The clinician can avoid conducting biased evaluations that merely serve to confirm preconceived ideas about a child by carefully testing *each* hypothesis. The Hypothesis Generation and Testing Worksheet can be helpful in this regard (see Appendix A). By developing a specific evaluation plan for each hypothesis and recording supporting and refuting evidence for each hypothesis as it is obtained, the clinician can easily organize the evaluation process, as well as make sure that no hypotheses are overlooked. The Hypothesis Generation and Testing Worksheet also can help in supervision (one can review the trainee's evaluation plan to check for omissions) or in consultation with colleagues on challenging cases.

Testing Hypotheses Regarding Physical Contributors to the Child's Pain

The Pain Medication History or Medication Record

To test this hypothesis, one must know exactly what pain medication the child has been *prescribed*, and then ascertain what exactly the child is *receiving*. The two may not be identical. In an inpatient setting, a good starting point is the medical chart and nursing records. Any pain medications prescribed should be noted in a physician's orders, which should include the dose and schedule of administration. For example, Mary may be prescribed "500 mg Tylenol® #3, q6, p.r.n." This means she should receive 500 mg of Tylenol® #3 (which contains codeine, a narcotic pain reliever) every 6 hours *as needed*.

Familiarity with basic terminology used in prescriptions is helpful in interpreting medical charts. A comprehensive medical dictionary is a good reference for Latin terms typically used in prescriptions. (See Table 8.1.) The clinician should note the date the prescription was originally ordered and then follow along in the orders to see if any other medications presumed to affect pain have been added to the regimen. For example, antidepressants sometimes are used in combination with other analgesics. The prescription orders should also indicate if a prescription has been discontinued (e.g., "DC Tylenol® #3") or if a dose has been increased. A detailed chronology of most of the child's medications over the past several weeks can serve as a useful reference point for testing a variety of hypotheses regarding pain medications.

The clinician should also have a general knowledge of the recommended means of administering various medications and the possible side effects of the medications in order to recognize when children may be taking medications inap-

Table 8.1. Common Prescription Terms

Term	Definition
b.i.d.	twice a day
h.s.	at night
p.o.	by mouth
p.r.n.	as needed
q. 4	every 4 hours
q.d.	every day
q.i.d.	four times a day
t.i.d.	three times a day

propriately. For example, some medications cause stomach upset unless taken with food. The *Physician's Desk Reference* (PDR) is published annually and includes comprehensive listings of all medications, chemical structure, indications, and side effects. Organized both by trade names and by generic names, the PDR allows one to look up an unfamiliar drug and quickly determine its typical uses, how it is presumed to work, and the side effects or complications that may be associated with the medication.

Nursing records should indicate when the child actually was given medications. In most hospitals, nurses are required to witness the actual administration of the child's medication and note the time in a special log. If the child is being seen on an outpatient basis, the physician can be contacted (with the parent's permission) to review the chart and summarize the child's medication.

A Word of Caution

It is essential to keep in mind that this is the data collection, hypothesis testing stage only. Debates or discussions of the relative merits of various medications are not appropriate at this point and may actually severely jeopardize a working relationship with the medical team. The clinician must remain sensitive to the boundaries of psychological practice and medical practice. Anything that implies criticism of the practice of medicine should be avoided. Once a complete conceptualization has been developed, other options for medication management may be diplomatically explored with the child's physician.

ARE MEDICATIONS THAT ARE LIKELY TO HELP THE CHILD'S PAIN NOT BEING USED?

The sources of information to test this hypothesis include the medication history (from chart review or physician interview), an interview with the child's caregivers, an ongoing record of medications administered, and direct observations of the child. For a chronic pain problem, the relationship between the administration of the pain medication and the child's pain symptoms should be examined to see if the medication is offering satisfactory relief. For acutely painful medical procedures, the medication history or direct observation should show what analgesics, if any, have been used, and the degree of pain relief obtained. Data collected must be precise. For example, Tylenol® comes in a nonprescription strength as well as in stronger (prescription only) combinations with codeine.

It would be helpful to understand the current philosophy of the medical environment regarding pain medications. Do they treat many children with pain problems? Do they have a pediatric anesthesiologist available to consult? Do they routinely use analgesics in this clinic? Have they had bad experiences in the past with pain medications?

ARE PAIN MEDICATIONS BEING ADMINISTERED INAPPROPRIATELY OR IN A LESS THAN IDEAL MANNER?

To test this hypothesis one needs to know three things: (1) how the medication currently is prescribed—at what dose, and when and how it is to be administered; (2) exactly when the child actually received the pain medications and whether there were any difficulties administering the medication; and (3) the child's pain prior to and after receiving the medication. The medical chart or pain medication record will provide information regarding the first question. The remaining questions can be answered by observation of the child in the pain situation, and from the parent's and the child's pain diaries. Since this hypothesis involves timing, accurate timing of observations of the child's pain experience is crucial.

Inappropriate Dose

Observation, interviews, or pain records can be used to determine if the child initially appeared to benefit from the medication but no longer seems to experience the same level of relief. If the child's weight has changed in the interim, a dose adjustment may be necessary. If the child's size has not changed and the pain medication has been used regularly, the possibility of tolerance should be considered. Finally, the PDR or a pharmacist can help determine if it might be possible to use higher doses of the current medication.

Inappropriate Timing or Scheduling

If the child is experiencing relatively constant pain, as would be expected in recovery from surgery, in a sickle cell pain crisis, or with pain secondary to a malignancy, the goal of medication should be to maintain a relatively constant state of comfort. Optimal comfort will allow the child to engage in rehabilitation activities and get much-needed sleep. A p.r.n. administration schedule usually is not appropriate in this situation. By definition, p.r.n. pain schedules require the child to first experience pain before being able to get the pain medication.

If pain medication is appropriately prescribed on an around-the-clock-basis, the pain administration records should be examined to determine if the child is actually provided the pain medication at the appropriate times. If the medication is administered on time, on a 6-hour schedule, for example, the pain records should be examined to see whether the child initially experiences relief from the medication and then re-experiences pain as the time of the next dose draws near. Some re-emergence of discomfort may be unavoidable, but the child should not be experiencing high levels of pain during the last hour or two before receiving the next dose of medication (or before the next dose takes effect). Such breakthrough pain increases the child's anxiety and guarantees that the subsequent dose will not be as effective in alleviating the pain.

Timing also is important in acute or intermittent pain situations. For example, pain administration records should be examined to determine if proper procedure was followed in administering analgesics prior to a painful procedure. To answer this question, one needs to know how long it takes for the medication to start working (and whether this depends on extraneous factors, such as whether or not the child had a full stomach), and how long the agent remains effective. For example, one patient was appropriately prescribed Tylenol® prior to painful physical therapy sessions. However, he erroneously took the medication as he walked into the physical therapy gym. By the time the medication could start working, his therapy session was half over and he was already miserable! In cases of headaches or other intermittent pain problems, the pain medication should be taken at the earliest signs of pain, so that it can begin to work while the pain is still manageable.

Administration Problems

Interviews conducted in a sensitive and accepting manner may reveal problems families may be experiencing in adhering to medication recommendations. Managing multiple medications on various schedules can be extremely difficult for patients. It is very important to communicate to families that it is OK to "confess" to missing doses of medications, since the goal is to try to make the process of administering the medication work better for the family. One should not assume that patients only forget to take prophylactic medications. Even medications designed to provide nearly immediate relief can be forgotten. For example, adolescent patients sometimes have difficulty getting organized enough in the morning to remember to take pain medications with them to school or work.

By acknowledging these difficulties up front, families may be more willing to report their actual compliance behaviors. For example, one can phrase a question in the following manner: "My patients tell me that it is really difficult to remember to keep all of these medications on hand at all times and even harder to remember to give them on time. One of my jobs is to try to come up with ways to make it easier for families to organize all of these details. What has it been like for you? When do you have the most trouble remembering to give your child her medications? What about yesterday, were you able to remember to give her any of the scheduled pain medications?"

Unstructured questioning, such as "Tell me about your day yesterday," may also reveal important contributors to adherence problems. Alternatively, the clinician could use the more structured 24-hour recall methodology frequently used in diet and diabetes adherence studies (e.g., Christensen, Terry, Wyatt, Pichert & Lorenz, 1983; Johnson, Silverstein, Rosenbloom, Carter, & Cunningham, 1986) to assess medication adherence. The 24-hour recall procedure asks the child (or parent) to recount the previous day's events, starting when he/she awoke and ending when he/she went to bed. The interviewer should record any pain episodes, and pain medications, and any other pain management efforts. After the entire day has been described, the interviewer should then ask specifically about the pain behaviors of interest (e.g., Did you take any prescription medications yesterday? Did you take any over-the-counter medications yesterday?). Studies using this methodology for diet and diabetes management emphasize the importance of conducting the interview in a nonjudgmental manner that allows patients to report their activities honestly. For diabetes management, Johnson et al. (1986) sampled two weekdays and one weekend day over a 2-week period by making unannounced telephone calls to the patients' homes (Johnson et al., 1986). A similar approach could be employed for pain medications as well as for a variety of other pain management behaviors.

The goal of the interview at this point in the assessment is to try to assess how many pain medication doses may be missed and what factors are contributing to these missed doses. For example, is the medication unavailable outside of the home? Does the child forget to take the medication before leaving for school? The clinician also can ask patients to record when they take their medications in conjunction with keeping a pain diary. One should keep in mind that this record keeping might, in itself, improve their compliance with the medications by serving as a reminder.

Forgetting is not the only reason for nonadherence with medication. Even if the parent remembers, if the child is not cooperative, it may be virtually impossible to get the medication into the child. Screaming, spitting, biting, and vomiting up the medication are common reactions of young children. At the end of such a battle, it is often difficult to determine how much, if any, of the medication was actually swallowed. Parent interview is a good starting point to identify the pattern of the child's resistance. Does the child protest all medications, or just this one? In what form is the medication given? Some pills are huge and dry and seem to stick to the tongue; others are tiny and slippery with no taste at all. Many medications are available in both liquid and tablet forms. How does the medication taste? Have the parents tried mixing the medication into any other substance to try to hide it or the flavor? Once the pattern of protest over ingestion is identified, one can try to estimate the volume of medication actually consumed. Record keeping might be more helpful at this point, since it is difficult to remember from time to time whether the child swallowed $\frac{1}{8}$ tsp or $\frac{1}{4}$ tsp medication on a given day. It may be helpful to give parents a set of measuring spoons to use to estimate how much medication the child received.

Misconceptions and Fears

Sensitive interviewing and obtaining the trust of the child and family are necessary to identify concerns that may be interfering with using the medication as prescribed. Few people will confront the doctor's authority outright if they have misgivings about a prescription. They are much more likely to simply throw the prescription away. In fact, it has been estimated that between 30 and 70 percent of patients do not comply with their physician's recommendations (Sacket & Haynes, 1976).

Again, a message of tolerance and acceptance is crucial to elicit this information. For example, questions can be prefaced with remarks such as: "There are pros and cons to using any medications. What are some of the disadvantages or negatives about using these medications from your point of view?" Or, "Many parents have concerns about over-relying on medications, especially strong medications, such as narcotics. What are the most important concerns for you?" Religious beliefs, participation in Alcoholics Anonymous (AA), or other chemical-free values may not be admitted in the initial interview. However, by approaching the discussion with an accepting and tolerant standpoint, one may help the child or family express their concerns later.

If a tolerant attitude is not conveyed, communication can quickly shut down, as the following example illustrates: A teenager who had successfully recovered from a very serious drug addiction was reluctant to take narcotic pain medications for a back injury, despite being physically very uncomfortable. She was following AA guidelines to remain "chemical-free," especially with respect to mind-altering substances. When her physician suggested using antidepressants in combination with pain medication, she attempted to bring up her concerns about psychoactive drugs. She perceived his response as insensitive: "So, just because it's called an antidepressant, you're going to get all bent out of shape about this?" Needless to say, she did not take the medication and did not further attempt to clarify her fears with her physician.

Even if addiction is not brought up as a concern, it may be advisable to introduce the topic to all families, in order to begin to educate them regarding real versus improbable addiction risks. Finally, specific fears regarding side effects of pain medications also should be assessed by interview. In particular both the child and the parents should be asked (separately) if the child has ever had any unpleasant side effects from medications, and if the child or parents have any concerns about possible side effects.

Unavailable Medication

It is extremely difficult to actually prove that someone else is using the child's medication, or that the medication is not being purchased. One can ask that the medication bottle be brought to the office and then check the prescription dates. If financial concerns are suspected, offering financial assistance through charitable organizations may broach the topic indirectly. The most convincing evidence that medications are not being given at home comes from dramatic changes in blood levels taken when medications are being managed by the family, and then comparing them with levels obtained when the child is admitted to the hospital and medications are managed by medical staff. The best that can be accomplished in such situations, unless the family confides their difficulties, is to identify the failure to receive medication doses and then address solutions to the problem that do not depend on family finances and do not allow someone other than the child access to the medication.

ARE OTHER PHYSICAL FACTORS EXACERBATING THE CHILD'S PAIN?

Protective Posturing

An interview with the parents or other adults in the environment can provide important information regarding the nature of any protective posturing. Often the protective position is the outward sign of the child's subjective pain experience that tells the adult that the child is in pain. For example, parents often notice limping or avoiding touching a body part, reluctance to walk or stand, and staying in bed. Pain diaries can then be used to identify the frequency and duration of these protective behaviors. One can also set up analog observations in order to directly observe the child walking, running, sitting at a desk, etc.

Fatigue

If inadequate sleep is a problem, children and families often do not realize it, unless inability to sleep is directly related to the pain problem itself. Therefore, it may not come up in interviews unless specifically assessed. Again, the clinician should avoid asking if the child "gets enough sleep." Rather, time in bed, time actually going to sleep (not necessarily even close to time going to bed), and time awakening should be determined. Children may be able to recall sleep information for a day or two. However, daily records may provide more accurate ongoing data. If the child's daily sleep is far less than normal for his/her age, fatigue may be exacerbating the pain situation. Daily records will also reveal whether the child's amount of sleep is age-appropriate but the sleep schedule is disrupted. For example, after a bad night with significant pain, a child may sleep most of the next day. It is easy, then, for the sleep cycle to get disrupted, resulting in the child being asleep during the day but being awake most of the night.

Disrupted sleep cycles are problematic for a number of reasons. Sleeping through the day prevents the child from engaging in age-appropriate activities. Furthermore, when one is awake at night, there generally are fewer stimuli available to distract from pain sensations. Thus, the experience of pain often is worst at night.

Environmental Variables

Some potentially interfering environmental factors can be identified through quick screening questions: Where do you sleep? Is the mattress soft or firm? How do you carry your books? Where do you sit to do your homework? How far is it from first period to second period class?

A physical therapy evaluation may be helpful in identifying appropriate limits regarding the child's strength and stamina as well as other aspects of the environment that may be interfering with the child's pain. For example, some backaches can be "cured" by switching from a briefcase to a backpack, or by adjusting the height of a chair.

Scheduling of Activities

Interviews with the child and adults in the environment can be used to determine whether the child takes appropriate breaks from physical activity or persists until unbearable pain makes him/her stop. If the child has been told to take rest breaks, asking directly, "Do you take rest breaks like your doctor told you to?" is likely to just encourage lying. Rather, the use of rest breaks can be evaluated by asking the child to recount a recent physical activity in a minute-by-minute fashion. One can then determine from the narrative whether rest breaks occurred at appropriate intervals. Similarly, narratives can be used to determine whether appropriate comfort measures (such as heat) were employed in preparation for physical activity.

9

Testing Hypotheses Regarding Cognitive and Emotional Contributors to the Child's Pain

As is true of any aspect of psychotherapy with children, it is often very difficult to obtain information regarding their underlying emotional experience. Young children, in particular, lack the cognitive ability to think about themselves objectively or to distinguish their thoughts and feelings from external events. For children under the age of 5 or 6, the main sources of information about the child's pain cognitions and emotions will come from direct observation of the child's behavior and from the observations of others in the environment. Older children may be able to provide some information regarding their experience via interviews, but even at older ages, direct observation often is the most helpful source of data.

IS THE CHILD'S ATTENTION FOCUSED ON THE PAIN?

Observing the child in the natural environment (e.g., in the classroom, or in a play activity, or while receiving a painful medical treatment) often will reveal the direction of the child's attention. If the child is sitting with his/her head down on the desk, there is little chance for distraction to help reduce the pain experience. If the child is staring at the needle and not talking to anyone or playing with anything, attention focus on the painful stimulus is pretty clear. The clinician should assess whether any potentially distracting activities are available in the environment as well as the percentage of time the child appears to be attending to sources of distraction versus the internal or external pain stimuli. Although one cannot know for certain what the child is actually concentrating on, one can at least infer attention from eye gaze, verbal interaction, and manipulation of toys or other objects. Assessment should also note whether adults attempt to engage the child in distracting activities, what specific activities are suggested, and how the child responds to these efforts. Does the child seems interested at first but tire of the activity, or does the activity seem uninteresting or developmentally inappropriate? Does the adult praise the child for engaging in the distracting activity and continue to prompt the child periodically, or does the adult expect the child to use the distraction activity independently?

The content of conversation during the pain episode will also provide information regarding the child's attention focus. If everyone is talking about pain— asking the child how he/she is feeling or trying to reassure the child that a shot will not hurt, the child's attention is being directed toward the pain stimulus. Adults often are unaware of the fact that they are inadvertently calling attention to pain in this manner.

For recurrent pain problems, direct observation may not be possible. Parent and child pain diaries may help pinpoint the child's attentional focus. For example, the clinician may look for the number of times per day the child mentions any pain-related sensations and the relative amount of time the child appears to spend focused on body sensations (i.e., "laying in bed listening to my stomach growl") versus the amount of time the child is engaged in adaptive behaviors unrelated to pain.

IS ANXIETY OR STRESS EXACERBATING THE CHILD'S PAIN?

Observation of the child often will reveal whether *aspects of the child's environment are frightening*. The child who cringes at the sight of the doctor or who starts to cry when entering the examination room may well be frightened. One should assume under most circumstances that the child will experience fear or anxiety if important adults are acting frightened or upset in his/her presence. The clinician should watch for crying, tears, grimacing, and other obvious signs of adult distress as well as the more subtle indicators, such as turning away or talking louder and more rapidly. For example, one youngster told his therapist that he knew things were "really bad" when his mother became "deadly calm." When she used an emotionless, extremely calm voice, he said he knew something was terribly wrong.

Interviews with the parent and medical personnel regarding exactly what the child has been told about the pain will reveal whether important information needed to make the pain understandable has been neglected. For example, a child experiencing phantom limb pain after an amputation thought she was being "haunted" by her lost leg until the concept of phantom pain was explained to her.

In acute pain situations, direct observation and interviews with parents will reveal whether *clear signals are lacking for the onset and termination of the painful stimulus*. A clear, unequivocal signal should immediately precede the painful injection or suture removal and an honest clear signal should indicate when the painful phase is over. Parents or staff may believe they are providing such signals, but observation may actually indicate that the signals are unclear. For example, in the course of a medical procedure, the child often is told, "we're done," even while the medical professional continues doing something to the child. From the child's standpoint, these doctors are *not* done.

Does the Pain Increase under Stressful Conditions?

Evidence for this hypothesis will come from the *pattern* of the child's pain over the course of the day and over the course of the week. The clinician may obtain the necessary information from interviews with the child, the parent, the child's teacher, or other school officials, such as the school nurse. However, unless the patterns are very obvious (e.g., the child who has pain every morning before school but at no other time), the clinician will probably also need to collect daily pain records. These records can then be analyzed to determine possible sources of stress in the child's environment. Follow-up interviews may then be helpful in identifying more precisely what about the setting is stressful for the child. For example, a pattern of pain complaints at lunch and at recess may emerge. Further interviews may reveal that the child is being teased by older children during recess and in the lunchroom. The child's frustration, anger, and dread of these social conflicts may be accompanied by increased pain.

Direct measurement of physiological responses to stress also can be used to test the hypothesis that stress plays a role in the child's pain. For example, as part of their evaluation of a 10-year-old migraine patient, O'Brien & Haynes (1995) measured heart rate, fingertip temperature, and fingertip blood flow during brief laboratory stress situations. (The stressor was subtracting serial 7s from 300 as quickly as possible.) Their patient developed a severe headache midway through the 4-minute stress period. At rest, she had an elevated heartrate and a low finger temperature. During the stressor, her heart rate and vasodilation increased; during the recovery period, she showed increasing vasoconstriction. Their results "supported the hypothesis that stress, combined with SNS [sympathetic nervous system] hypersensitivity and excessive vasoconstriction, was a powerful elicitor of migraine headaches" (p. 74).

DOES THE CHILD ENGAGE IN SELF-DEFEATING THINKING ABOUT THE PAIN?

Pain self-statements are unlikely to be captured in general questions or by interviews with other adults, because these thoughts tend to be "automatic"—the child probably is unaware of them. With older children, one can adapt general cognitive-behavioral assessment strategies (e.g., Kendall, 1991) to explore this issue through interview or daily pain diaries. With both methods, one should focus on a specific painful episode and try to get the child to report the thoughts or self-statements made as the event was occurring. For example, "Tell me about the pain you had this morning. When did the pain start? What did you think when you first noticed the pain? What thoughts went through your mind?" If the child is unable to provide an answer, one can suggest possibilities, such as: "Here are some thoughts other children have shared with me. See if any of these might be thoughts you had this morning. 'Hey, this is great! I get to stay home today!' 'Oh no, not again!' 'I can't take this!' 'I'm sick of hurting!' 'I'm never going to get better.' 'I can't take another day like yesterday.' 'Why does this have to happen to me? It's so unfair.' 'I'll never be able to pass my math test today with this pain!'" If the child will co-operate with daily pain diaries, the specific thoughts experienced at each pain re-cording point can then be written down and examined later to identify potentially self-defeating attitudes.

It may also be useful to administer a structured scale, such as the Coping Strategies Questionnaire for Sickle Cell Disease (Gil et al., 1991), to identify cop-ing strategies. The CSQ lists several different coping strategies, which children rate on a 7-point Likert scale to indicate how often they use them. It should be noted, however, that some children under the age of 9 may not understand how to use the Likert scaling (Dahlquist, 1990). Moreover, clinicians should be cautious in interpreting children's reports on any forced choice instrument. Because of their suggestibility, children may endorse items presented in this format that they would not report in an open-ended, unstructured format (Ross & Ross, 1988).

DOES THE PAIN HAVE SIGNIFICANT EMOTIONAL MEANING FOR THE CHILD?

This issue is difficult to assess in the beginning stages of a pain evaluation. A trust-ing therapeutic relationship usually is needed before children will confide serious fears or concerns. For example, leg pain in a child with cancer may be extremely frightening, since it may be a sign of relapse. The child or parent may be terrified that the child may die, making the pain much more difficult to handle. The thera-pist should remain open to this possibility, even if initial interviews with the child do not reveal serious concerns.

Parent interviews may also provide data regarding the emotional meaning of the pain for the child as well as for the parent. One mother confessed that she felt anxious days before her child's medical treatments because she knew she could do nothing to help him. She reported feeling stressed and even had bouts of diarrhea for days preceding each treatment. Observations of the parent–child interactions during the pain episode also provides information regarding emotional signifi-cance of the pain, although the exact nature of their emotions may need to be clari-fied by sensitive probing after the event. For example, the parent who sobs during the child's medical procedure may be feeling frustrated, incompetent, empathy for the child's pain, anger that the father did not come to help her, or grief related to the illness.

IS THE CAREGIVER'S EMOTIONAL OR COGNITIVE STATUS INTERFERING WITH HIS/HER ABILITY TO ASSIST THE CHILD IN MANAGING THE PAIN?

To test this hypothesis, the clinician must understand the family context in which the child's pain occurs. This requires a more general intake interview that evaluates stresses and resources within the family and community. Such interview data will provide evidence of factors that may be contributing to parental ineffectiveness. However, this premise also can be tested by direct observation of the parent's behavior. Parents who do not seem to understand what is involved in the child's medical regimen or frequently leave the child to attend to crises in their personal lives may not be able to provide the consistent assistance the child may need to manage the pain. The obvious implication for treatment, then, is finding another adult to assist the child.

Testing Hypotheses Regarding Behavioral Contributors to the Child's Pain

As outlined in Chapter 5, it is crucial to evaluate the factors that may be maintaining the child's pain behaviors as well as the factors that may be maintaining the parents' behaviors in their interaction with their child. We will consider the evaluation of parental behaviors and children's behavior separately, since different assessment strategies may be needed. We will begin with an examination of the contingencies that may maintain the child's pain behaviors.

THE CHILD'S PAIN BEHAVIORS AND PAIN COPING BEHAVIORS

To What Degree Is the Child's Pain Behavior Positively Reinforced?

Direct observation will provide the best information regarding the child's pain behaviors and the events that precede and follow these behaviors. If pain behaviors are of fairly high frequency, one can observe the child in the natural environment—in the hospital room, the clinic, in the classroom, or on the playground. If such observation can be conducted in an unobtrusive manner, one may be able to get an accurate picture of the child's pain behaviors. However, it is difficult to avoid problems of reactivity, even if unstructured observation is employed, and the clinician must always consider the possibility that the child's behavior is not representative of typical behavior when not being observed.

If the pain behaviors are infrequent, the clinician may want to structure the observation situation to increase the chances that the child's pain behaviors will be observed. For example, one can ask the child to engage in some sort of physical activity that is likely to be associated with some discomfort. For children who insist

Date: _____ Time:_____ Observer:_____
Setting: _____

A Antecedents (What happened first)	B Pain behaviors shown by the child	C Consequences (What happened next)

Figure 10.1. ABC pain chart.

on staying in bed to avoid pain, sitting up or walking may be appropriate activities to observe. If the pain involves medical procedures, one should observe the actual painful procedure or therapy session. Videotaping the observation session is very helpful, since it enables one to review the child's behavior multiple times in the process of identifying potential consequences of the child's behavior.

The observer should document any pain behaviors that occur as well as the events preceding and the events following the pain behaviors. A basic A-B-C (Antecedent–Behavior–Consequences) chart can be used to document the observed interactions. (See Figure 10.1.). The same format can be used by others in the child's environment as well. For example, the parents can record their observations of the child's pain behaviors at home; the teacher or nurse can record pain episodes as they occur in other settings, or the therapist may choose to observe the child. The observational record can then be examined to test the hypothesis that the child's pain behaviors are positively reinforced.

Consider the observational record obtained by an experienced therapist presented in Figure 10.2. In this example, the mother provides considerable attention to the child's pain behaviors. First, she appears to interpret a behavior that may simply have been one of disagreement or irritability as indicative of pain. Then, she attends to the child's groans, whimpers, and eventual pain verbalizations both verbally and by physically stroking her.

A Antecedents (What happened first)	B Pain behaviors shown by the child	C Consequences (What happened next)
Sally was watching TV sitting in bed. No apparent distress. Mom said, "It's time to get up and get ready for PT, honey."		
	Sally groans, grimaces, does not shift position.	Mom: "What's the matter, don't you feel well?"
	Sally groans louder and whines: "No!"	Mom: "Is it your head? Does your head hurt?"
	Sally: "Yes, my head and my tummy hurt." Starts to whimper.	Mom: "Do you want me to rub your tummy?" Begins to rub Sally's abdomen while Sally continues to whimper softly. Still watching TV.
Mom gets up, goes to phone	Sally whimpers more loudly, starts to cry.	Mom: "I'm not going anywhere, honey. I'm just calling your nurse. Maybe you don't need to go to PT right now. You just rest."
Mom calls nurse, tells her Sally is hurting too much to go to PT. Requests Tylenol®.	Sally whimpers quietly in bed.	Nurse comes in, gives Sally Tylenol®. Mom sits in bed beside Sally.

Figure 10.2. Behavioral observations of a 4-year-old girl recovering from surgery.

Of course, not all behavioral observations will be this clear-cut. The most complete picture of the contingencies affecting the child's pain behaviors will be obtained if several pain episodes are observed and if observations are conducted in multiple settings by multiple observers. This allows the clinician to identify *patterns* of behavior and consequences in addition to single episodes, which is crucial in cases of intermittent reinforcement of pain behavior. The clinician should keep in mind that inconsistencies may emerge *within* an individual (e.g., sometimes attending to pain behavior and other times ignoring it) or *between* individuals (e.g., the mother may be firm and consistent in enforcing physical therapy exercises despite the child's pain, while the father may be more variable in his requirements, depending on how the child feels at the moment). The length of time one should monitor pain behaviors will depend on the frequency of pain behaviors (contingencies may be easier to identify when the behavior occurs more frequently) and the degree of variability in the behavior and in the environmental consequences (it may take longer to identify patterns if the behavior or consequences are highly variable).

Interview data alone also can provide information regarding ongoing contingencies. For example, the parent, child, or teacher may be asked to describe a recent pain episode in detail and describe the sequence of events leading up to and following the child's pain behavior. However, such retrospective recall can be inaccurate and should be used cautiously. Parents may forget what happened, or they may not be very good at objectively reporting their own behavior. Parents often claim that they "ignored" their child's misbehavior when in reality they paid considerable attention to the misbehavior. By having parents or others monitor pain behaviors as they occur, and then discussing the records, some of the problems inherent in retrospective recall can be avoided.

The importance of peers as sources of positive reinforcement for pain behaviors should not be overlooked. One 14-year-old patient refused to get out of his wheelchair, despite his excellent strength and endurance. It took several interviews before he revealed that he was being pushed around the school in his wheelchair by a compassionate (and attractive) female classmate who had volunteered to help handicapped students. He had never received so much attention from an attractive girl before. Thus, he was uninterested in making any behavioral changes that would jeopardize his new-found status.

To What Degree Is the Child's Pain Behavior Negatively Reinforced?

The same sources of data—behavioral observations and self-monitoring—can be used to identify possible negative reinforcement of pain behavior. Avoidance of unpleasant tasks, avoidance of emotionally stressful situations, and avoidance of increased pain (real or anticipated) are some common examples of negative reinforcement of pain behaviors in children. Negative reinforcement often occurs in combination with other positive reinforcement contingencies. To illustrate, let us return to the interaction between Sally and her mother introduced in Figure 10.2.

In addition to providing considerable attention to Sally's pain behaviors, her mother also cancels her physical therapy session because of her pain. Thus, Sally avoids the uncomfortable physical therapy exercises. Groaning, whimpering, crying, and pain verbalizations are negatively reinforced by avoiding the unpleasant physical therapy situation.

Physical therapy is easily identified as a noxious experience. Physical therapy exercises are often uncomfortable or actually painful. The avoidance of the unpleasant stimulus was easy to identify in this example. However, in many cases, one may need to really get to know a child before the aversive situations can be identified. For example, one high school patient was too short to sit at the benches and worktables in his auto shop class. Furthermore, he was the only overweight, unathletic teen in his section, and he felt like he was surrounded by "jocks" and tough kids. He was terrified that the other boys were going to tease him for needing a taller chair and was too mortified to ask the teacher to help him solve the problem. It took him weeks to confess that this was his fear. In the interim, he was successfully avoiding this class by staying home from school because of his "severe" pain complaints.

To What Degree Is Pain Coping Behavior Inadequately Reinforced or Actually Punished?

If pain behavior is serving some function for the child, there is a good chance that the positive behaviors we would like the child to engage in might come at some cost to the child. The child who loses attention from a busy parent when pain-free is unlikely to want to stop complaining of pain. The child who is ridiculed at school for using relaxation exercises is not likely to continue pain coping efforts. Thus it also is important to examine what happens when the child is pain-free or when the child engages in behaviors designed to reduce pain.

The format of data collection can parallel the format used to identify pain behaviors. Direct observation and recording conducted by the clinician and others in the child's environment and clinical interviews can be employed. However, defining the target behavior being observed is more difficult. It is easier to record instances in which a behavior occurs (e.g., the child screams, or the child takes a slow relaxing breath) than it is to record instances involving the *absence* of a behavior. Thus, the clinician needs to develop a clear operational definition of the desired behaviors—the behaviors the child *should* demonstrate. Examples of target behaviors that may be helpful to monitor include school attendance, participation in physical education class, on-time arrival in class, time out of bed, interactions with peers, walking (distance or duration), clothes put on independently, cheerful voice tone, quiet (moan-free) resting, sleep, and duration of play with peers. Observing the antecedents and consequences of these desirable behaviors should reveal whether the rewards for the behaviors are inadequate, which is very common, and may indicate subtle ways in which pain coping behaviors may be punished.

Does the Child Lack the Skills Necessary to Perform the Adaptive Behavior(s)?

Cognitive and Academic Deficits

The ways in which cognitive deficits, learning disabilities, and academic deficits can be evaluated are the same as those used in general child clinical practice. Although it is not efficient to conduct a full psychoeducational battery with every child, clinicians should keep in mind that subtle academic difficulties are very common in otherwise bright children experiencing pain symptoms that result in school absence. For example, many children who have pain problems report that they enjoy school, like their teachers, have many friends, and have a history of good grades. Psychoeducational testing sometimes later reveals that several of these stomach pain and headache sufferers have mild deficits in one particular academic area. Because they were very bright, they had been able to compensate for their deficits to some degree, but were experiencing considerable stress in the process. For example, one boy had such poor spelling skills that he could barely write a readable sentence. However, he was able to compensate by using the spell check on his home computer. No one was aware of his problem. His teacher merely assumed he was doing sloppy work when he turned in misspellings. His stomach aches kept him home from school and enabled him to use the computer for almost all of his make-up work, thus avoiding the embarrassment of his poor spelling.

Social and Communication Skills Deficits

Another child had been ill for so long and had missed so much school that he had failed to learn very basic "survival" skills for interactions with peers. For example, although he could talk at length with adults, he did not know how to start up a conversation with a child he didn't know well or how to join a group already playing together. He had no conflict resolution skills and had no idea how to respond to threats or teasing from peers. Given these serious skill deficits, the chances of this boy experiencing positive reinforcement in the school setting were very low. Thus it is not surprising that he continued to complain of pain in order to avoid going to school, even when his disease was in remission.

Social skill deficits, especially deficits specific to peer interactions, may not be readily apparent in an interview with the child. The parent may not realize the extent of the child's difficulties either. These deficits may be masked if the child spends a lot of time with adults or with one particular friend or with a restricted circle of companions (e.g., other chronically ill children). Although precise norms for the number of friends appropriate at a specific age or the number of extracurricular activities appropriate for children with chronic illnesses are lacking, there are some general signs one can look for as indicators of potential problems. For example, children who rarely spend time with peers or only socialize with younger peers or with family members may have skill deficits. Screening instruments such as the Socialization and Daily Living Subscales of the Vineland Adaptive Behavior Scales (Sparrow, Balla, & Cicchetti, 1984) or the Peer Interaction Record (PIR) (Thompson, Power, & Dahlquist, 1994) can help identify children who may need further evaluation.

To specifically assess social and communication skills, observation of the child in actual interactions with peers or family members is warranted. If observations in the natural environment are not feasible, analog situations can be created in the therapist's office. For example, one can role-play a situation involving teasing from peers and see how the child responds. Family members can be observed discussing a problem or making a decision to reveal maladaptive communication skills.

The child's ability to express himself/herself emotionally can be observed in day-to-day interactions and also assessed in an interview with the child. Is the child able to label feelings appropriately? Can he/she identify a variety of emotional states? Can he/she distinguish pain states from other affective states?

ADULT RESPONSES TO THE CHILD

In the process of observing the child, the clinician can begin to identify facilitating and hindering behaviors on the part of the parent, medical personnel, or other adults in the environment and then test hypotheses regarding the contingencies that may be maintaining the adults' behavior (in addition to examining contingencies affecting the child's behavior). Many of the consequences important in maintaining the adults' behaviors may occur outside of the interaction with the child or may be difficult to observe. Therefore, interviews with the adults should be included in addition to direct observations. The hypotheses tested in the following section address the *function* that the adults' behavior toward the child may play in their life.

To What Degree Is the Adult's Problematic Behavior Positively Reinforced?

Many adults will acknowledge when interviewed that it can feel deeply satisfying to cuddle and comfort a hurting child. They may feel a strong sense of competence and effectiveness after successfully "fixing" a youngster's discomfort. The appreciation and desire for the adult's presence may be especially rewarding to the parent of an otherwise independent child who may not need his parent's ministrations very often.

Direct observation may also reveal attention or other positive interactions with others that may serve to reinforce the parent's behavior with the child. For example, parental attention to pain behaviors often appears to be followed by attention from medical staff. The attention may be specific in content and related to the child's illness, or it may center on nonmedical content. For example, one mother of a child was informally observed in the clinic while her daughter's pain complaints were being evaluated. After a few visits, it became apparent that the mother's primary adult social interactions occurred in the clinic. She lived in an isolated setting and had little money for entertainment or even transportation. However, when her child was in pain, she could justify the trip to the medical center, where she had the opportunity to socialize with many parents as well as concerned, sympathetic health care providers. In many ways, the medical clinic became one of the most enjoyable settings in her life.

To What Degree Is the Adult's Problematic Behavior Negatively Reinforced?

In almost all cases, the adult's responses are to some degree negatively reinforced by a change in some aspect of the child's aversive or unpleasant behavior. For example, direct observation will reveal whether the child stops complaining of pain or complains less intensely after the parent rubs her back. One may observe that the child stops crying in protest as soon as the parent stops pushing him to get out of bed or stops pressuring him to get dressed. In these observations the reciprocity involved in pain interactions becomes apparent, as parents inadvertently teach their children pain behaviors and children inadvertently teach their parents to give in to their protests.

It is also important to explore other consequences of parent–child pain interactions that also may function to negatively reinforce parental pain management strategies. For example, parents who are able to avoid unpleasant work situations by staying home with their sick child may have little incentive to see their child's pain remit. Focusing undue attention on the child's pain complaints may allow the parent to avoid unpleasant conflicts with the spouse. Testing these hypotheses may require several interviews with the parents in which the therapist explores the quality of other aspects of their lives and the impact of the child's pain behavior on the stressful or unpleasant aspects of their life, in particular.

To What Degree Is Appropriate Adult Behavior Punished or Inadequately Reinforced?

In families with high levels of conflict, one often will see examples of actual punishment for appropriate efforts to deal with the child's pain during direct observation. One of the parents will criticize the other, for example, for being too hard on the child. Given that many parents feel guilty when being firm and pushing their child when the child has pain, despite being told by the physician that they should do so, this criticism can quickly undercut their efforts to continue setting firm goals for pain coping behaviors. Even in the midst of learning pain management strategies, we have observed parents comment on how ineffective the other parent is in managing the child's pain or brag about how much better the child did with them than with the other parent. It's quite understandable that the criticized parent would feel punished for his/her efforts to deal appropriately with the child's pain and just give up.

If the important family members are not available to be observed, or if the conflicts are not as overt, parent interviews may reveal the ways in which appropriate parent behavior may be punished. For example, one mother of a child with arthritis was struggling to help her 12-year-old son get himself dressed every morning ánd walk to the bus stop despite his morning aches and stiffness. However, because of her work schedule, the son spent two days a week at his grandmother's house. On those days, his grandmother dressed him completely and wheeled him to the bus stop in a wheelchair. She complained daily to the boy that his mother was cruel to ignore his pain and called the mother at work each day to tell her how sick the poor boy was that day. The more the mother tried to enforce developmentally appropriate self-care goals for the boy, the more criticism she received from her mother-in-law. She certainly felt that her pain management efforts were punished by her mother-in-law. An effective pain management intervention for this family, therefore, would require a change in the grandmother's behavior or a change in the child care arrangements so that the grandmother could not sabotage the program.

Punishment can also come from the child. Younger children may hit, scream, throw tantrums, physically struggle, and tell parents they hate them in response to unwanted parental pain interventions. (One frustrated youngster told her parents she'd "never visit them in the nursing home when they got old…" if they didn't help her get dressed.) The child may keep parents awake most of the night with calls for assistance. If the parents have been inconsistent in their responses in the past (which most often is the case), this child behavior may last a long time and be quite intense. Direct observation and interviews in which the details of difficult interactions with the child are discussed may reveal these contingencies. Examination of the A-B-C pain records may also suggest ways in which the child's behavior serves to punish the parent's efforts.

With respect to positive reinforcement for appropriate behavior management of the child's pain, it is extremely rare that parents receive encouragement or recognition for what they are doing correctly. One should watch for such praise or encouragement in direct observation and probe for it in interviews and when reviewing parental reports of pain episodes. One should also assess potential sources of such positive reinforcement for the parents that could be incorporated into future clinical intervention.

── CASE EXAMPLE

In Figure 10.3, the parents of an 11-year-old girl (Jennifer), who was referred for chronic pain and poor school attendance, describe her pain behaviors over the course of a weekend. The first example describes some of Jennifer's pain behaviors, which primarily consisted of complaints that she hurt and requests for assis-

...ts d first)	B Pain behaviors shown by the child	C Consequences (What happened next)
Friday night We told her it was bedtime and she was to sleep in her bed. She said she didn't feel good. (Earlier in the day she fell on her foot getting out of the car.) She said her foot hurt and she could not walk. We told her to get in her bed. Jim finally put her in her bed.	She began to cry and yell, "I need help, I don't feel good." She asked us to call her doctor. She said she could not lie down. She kept screaming, "I hurt, somebody help me."	Finally at 10:20 PM I called the doctor and he told me to tell her she would be fine and to go to sleep. So we just left her in there and she finally went to sleep.
Saturday Since one of her heels hurts her she had several socks on to help and she slipped out of the car and bumped it again. Later in the day she slipped on the kitchen floor and said she needed help getting up. We told her she could get up by herself.	She kept laying there saying "I need help," over and over. Then she yelled, "Somebody help me!" We just sat there. We told her when we went out for ice cream we would just lock the door and leave her there if she couldn't get up.	Finally she managed to get up because she didn't want to be left.
Saturday night When we got back from having ice cream she said her foot was hurting and she needed help. We told her she could make it. So we came in and left her outside while she was complaining. It was very cold outside. Once we got inside, she began to scream.	She was screaming, "Help me, help me, somebody help me."	Jim opened the door and she was on the ground and he brought her in because I didn't want her to get too cold. If it had not been so cold we would have left her outside.

Figure 10.3. Behavioral records completed by the parents of an 11-year-old girl.

tance from her parents. It is apparent right away that the parents are inconsistent in their response to these behaviors. At first, the father reinforces her pain complaints and requests for assistance by putting her to bed. This could be conceptualized as positive reinforcement (help and attention) for pain complaints, as well as negative reinforcement (since her father carried her to bed, it allowed her to avoid the physical discomfort of walking to bed unassisted). Then, her pain complaints and yells escalate as the parents try not to respond to them. (In the past, her mother had slept with Jennifer whenever she was uncomfortable, but now the parents had resolved to stop sleeping with her at night.) Jennifer's behavior is a classic example of an extinction burst in response to the parents' termination of the previous positive reinforcement contingencies. Although it is not written in their record, when we discussed these data in the therapy session, the parents revealed that there was considerable conversation going on between the parents and Jennifer about her pain and her need to go to sleep by herself during this time period. Thus, the parents' attention probably intermittently positively reinforced Jennifer's complaints. Ultimately, the parents were able to ignore Jennifer's continued protests, and she eventually went to sleep.

In the next episode, Jennifer appears to be using a misguided technique to reduce her foot pain (putting several socks on), and this intervention only serves to make her more prone to slip and fall. When she falls, she requests help getting up, and her parents appropriately tell her she is capable of getting up unassisted and refuse to provide the unnecessary assistance. They report "just sitting there," but further questioning later revealed that they did converse with her extensively. Jennifer did eventually get up unassisted when it became clear that her parents were not going to help her and that she would lose access to a positive event if she did not comply. Thus, her protests were intermittently reinforced by parental attention, although her actual demands for assistance were not reinforced. The attention may have communicated a mixed message to Jennifer regarding whether or not her parents were going to remain firm in requiring her to help herself.

In the final episode recorded, Jennifer again demands assistance in a task her parents feel she can accomplish independently, namely getting out of the car. They initially do not respond and go into the house. She responds with escalating screams for assistance (an extinction burst). The parents respond by carrying her into the house, thus reinforcing her more intense protest behaviors.

The pain records presented in Figure 10.3 also suggest that reinforcement contingencies may be affecting the parents. First, Jennifer's screams take place in a highly public setting—in the front yard. Her screams would be readily heard by the neighbors. Continuing to ignore Jennifer's behavior has a high probability of causing embarrassment and maybe other negative events, such as neighbors calling the police. Thus, the parents' efforts to respond appropriately are followed by punitive consequences—feelings of embarrassment and anticipated negative social consequences. By carrying her into the house, they terminate her screams, which serves to negatively reinforce their behavior. The mother's narrative also hints at another negative consequence of her initial attempts to deal with the child appropriately—"If it had not been so cold, we would have left her outside." Although this may well have simply been a rationalization for her decision, it also suggests possible feelings of guilt, which may also function as a negative consequence of the parents' efforts to appropriately extinguish the child's pain behaviors.

Excerpts from the therapist's hypothesis generation and planning worksheet are presented in Figure 10.4.

Behavioral hypotheses	Sources of Data	Evaluation Plan	Test Results
A. *Is the child's pain behavior positively reinforced?*	Home observation School observation Clinic observation Jennifer's pain diary Parent pain records Teacher pain records Parental interview Interview Jennifer Teacher interview Counselor interview	1. Parental pain records 2. Parental interview Do later (if needed): • Teacher interview • School nurse interview • School observation	A. *Supported* (1 & 2) J's pain complaints are intermittently reinforced by extensive attention from both parents. Attention consists of conversation, explanation, arguing. (1 & 2) J's demands intermittently result in assistance from parents
B. *Is the child's pain behavior negatively reinforced?*	Same as A.	1. Parental pain records 2. Parental interview Do later (if needed): • Teacher interview • School nurse interview • School observation	B. *Supported* (1 & 2) J avoids having to walk, get up when she falls. (2) History of avoiding sleeping alone and helping herself at night by complaining of pain (1 & 2) Negative reinforcement is inconsistent. Parents try not to give in, but often eventually do.
C. *Is adaptive behavior inadequately reinforced or punished?*	Same as A	1. Parental pain records 2. Parental interview Do later (if needed): • Teacher interview • School nurse interview • School observation	C. *Unclear, insufficient data. Possible* (1) No reinforcement after J eventually slept in bed alone. (2) Did take child for ice cream after got up off the floor. Still don't know if there are negative consequences when Jennifer actually behaves appropriately. Plan: assess next session in interview with parents

Hypothesis	Assessment methods	Procedures	Findings
D. Does the child lack the skills necessary to perform the adaptive behavior? • Cognitive/academic deficits? • Social/communication deficits?	Intelligence tests Achievement tests Neuropsychological tests Interview with child Parent interview Teacher interview Counselor interview Observe at school & home	1. WISC-R 2. Woodcock–Johnson Achievement Test 3. Child interview 4. Teacher interview	D. Pending
E. Is the adult's problematic behavior positively reinforced?	Home, clinic observation Jennifer's pain diary Parent pain records Parent interview Interview with Jennifer Medical staff interview	1. Parental pain records 2. Parental interview Do later, if needed: • Home, clinic observation • Medical staff interview	E. No data yet
F. Is the adult's problematic behavior negatively reinforced?	Same as E	1. Parental pain records 2. Parent interview Later, if needed: • Home, clinic observation • Medical staff interview	F. Supported (1) Giving in terminates J's noxious behavior, decreases embarrassment, risk of police or other officials being called, reduces parental guilt (2) Evidence of parental guilt re: not helping J if she is in pain
G. Is appropriate adult behavior inadequately reinforced or punished?	Same as E	1. Parental pain records 2. Parental interview Later, if needed: • Home, clinic observation • Medical staff interview	G. No evidence yet Plan: ask about reactions of others to parents' new efforts to set limits on pain behaviors in next session.

Figure 10.4. Excerpts from Jennifer's hypothesis generation and evaluation planning worksheet.

11

Treating Physical Contributors to the Child's Pain

The appropriate pain management intervention should be readily apparent from the completed conceptualization. Any hypothesis that appears to have support should be addressed in the treatment plan. Thus, it should be possible to address multiple objectives within a single treatment plan. If it is too complex to address all components simultaneously, sets of treatment objectives should be prioritized, beginning with interventions that can serve as stepping stones to future gains. For instance, making sure the child is receiving appropriate pain medication should take precedence over beginning to teach psychological pain management strategies. Eliminating fears based on misconceptions and misinformation should take precedence over developing a reinforcement program in most cases. The Treatment Planning Worksheet provided in Appendix B may be photocopied and used to assist the clinician in organizing an appropriate treatment plan.

Under most circumstances, it is advisable to address physical hypotheses first in the treatment plan. The primary reason for this top prioritization is to avoid unnecessary pain. The data accumulated in the process of testing the physical hypotheses should indicate the physical contributors to the child's pain that should become the targets of intervention.

The next step involves specifying how each supported hypothesis can be treated and then prioritizing the components of the treatment plan. As can be seen in the following chapters, treatments based on the confirmed hypotheses often are very straightforward (in the case of changing a medication schedule). However, there may be many possible ways to treat a confirmed hypothesis, and these alternatives should be considered.

Many different components can be integrated into a single treatment plan. For example, intervention might include helping a child develop more appropriate rest breaks during exercise, applying warm heat before exercise, and taking Tylenol® 30 minutes before exercise. General guidelines for treating physical contributors to the child's pain are presented in Table 11.1.

Table 11.1. General Guidelines for Treating Physical Contributors to the Child's Pain

- Recommend a more effective pain management regimen
  - Recommend using a stronger or different medication
  - Recommend considering a change in the dosage of the pain medication
  - Recommend adjusting medication administration schedules
- Help the child and family better adhere to the prescribed medication regimen
  - Provide a structure for medication administration
  - Provide a more palatable form of medication
  - Address misconceptions and fears
- Make sure medications are available
- Help the child avoid protective posturing
- Improve the child's sleep patterns
- Modify environmental variables that exacerbate pain
- Schedule physical activities appropriately

PROBLEM: THE CHILD IS RECEIVING LESS THAN OPTIMAL PAIN MEDICATION

The specific treatment that should be implemented will depend on the way in which the child's pain medication currently is administered.

Recommend Consideration of a Stronger or Different Medication

If the medications likely to reduce the child's pain are not being used, the issue should be discussed with the child's physician to determine if alternative medications might be of benefit. There may well be a contraindication for using other pain medications. For example, cardiac or respiratory problems limit the types of pain medications a child can safely use. The discussion of alternative medications (and any other medically related issues) must be broached diplomatically and with respect for and acceptance of the fact that the physician (and not the mental health professional) is responsible for the child's medical care.

To avoid misunderstandings, it is essential to establish a good working relationship with the medical team. The groundwork for such a relationship begins when the clinician discusses the case early on with the child's physician. By obtaining information during the hypothesis testing phase, the clinician sets the stage for a team effort in understanding and treating the child's pain problem. Understanding the medical system can also make it easier to discuss medication alternatives with medical colleagues. For example, in a general medical setting where few children are treated, it might be appropriate to informally educate staff about the benefits of new topical anesthetics, such as EMLA®. In an academic medicine tertiary care setting, providing relevant research literature regarding medication options may be appropriate. For additional guidelines on developing effective consulting relationships with pediatricians see Drotar's (1995) comprehensive text.

Recommend Considering a Change in the Dosage of the Pain Medication

If the data suggest that a formerly effective pain agent is no longer effective, the pattern of data can be shared with the physician along with the clinician's impressions of why the dose no longer is effective (e.g., the child has gained weight since the initial prescription). Pointing out evidence of tolerance to the medication can also be helpful in assisting the physician in adjusting medication levels. Similarly, if the current dose is conservative, the clinician can diplomatically inquire about the possibility of increasing the dose.

Recommend Adjusting Medication Administration Schedules

In most cases of acute postsurgical pain, severe disease pain, and chronic unremitting pain, it is likely to be appropriate to recommend that the child be switched from a p.r.n. medication schedule to an around-the-clock schedule (McGrath, 1990). In episodic pain, such as recurrent headaches or recurrent abdominal pain, the pain may be unpredictable and occur at intervals of several days or weeks. It would not be appropriate to recommend around-the-clock pain medication between the pain episodes.

Providing a copy of a relevant article to put in the medical chart (especially in teaching hospitals) can be useful as an adjunct to scheduling recommendations. (For example, the U.S. Department of Health and Human Services has published clinical practice guidelines for acute pain management that summarize many of the principles discussed in this text. See the Recommended Readings more information on this and related publications.) To combat breakthrough pain, a shorter interval between pain administrations may be recommended for consideration. Again, by sharing the pain records with the physician, the clinician may provide extremely valuable information that will enable the physician to schedule the medications more effectively. For example, it may not be safe to give the current medication at shorter intervals. But, it may be possible to add another medication or stagger the scheduling of adjunctive medications, such as acetaminophen, to minimize breakthrough pain.

Patient-controlled analgesia (PCA) is another approach to optimizing pain medication delivery that is used primarily for intravenous drug administration after surgery or in severe cancer pain. PCA allows the patient to receive a certain amount of extra pain medication at preprogrammed intervals by pushing a button connected to the medication infusion system. Studies have found that children understand the PCA system and that they often achieve better pain control and use less of the medication overall with PCA than with standard administrations of the same drugs (McGrath, 1990). PCA also may have a secondary benefit of anxiety reduction, since the patient controls the access to the medication.

If it is more effective to administer pain medications at a specific time, the physician may be asked to write orders stating that explicitly. For example, the teenager who frequently forgot to ask for his p.r.n. pain medications before physical therapy did very well when his pain medications were ordered for 10:00 A.M. and 1:30 P.M., which was approximately 30 minutes prior to his morning and afternoon therapy sessions.

If family members are confused about the purpose of medications, the physician may be asked to explain again the purpose of the medication and why it is important to administer it in a certain way. Prescriptions can be written in such a way that the reason for administration is clearly specified (e.g., "take every morning to prevent inflammation" instead of merely "take every morning") to remind patients and parents. If a medication needs to reach a certain level in the blood before it will be effective, patients should be told this, so they will not stop taking the medication when it doesn't immediately relieve their pain. Clearly specifying when to stop certain medications also helps clear up confusion regarding symptomatic versus prophylactic medications.

Help the Child and Family Better Adhere to the Prescribed Medication Regimen

All the ways in which adherence can be improved cannot be addressed here. Indeed, entire books have been written on the topic. Meichenbaum and Turk's (1987) excellent text on facilitating treatment adherence is a useful guide for a wide range of adherence enhancing strategies. Some of the common adherence problems encountered with children receiving pain medications are addressed below.

Provide a Structure for Medication Administration

Pair the medications with an activity that the child or parent is not likely to forget. For example, medications can be paired with activities that always occur, such as getting up, eating lunch, and going to bed. If this pairing is done consistently (i.e., in the same manner every day), taking the medication will become associated with this event. Over time, the event will serve as a cue or reminder to take the medication. This process is called stimulus control. For example, one teen decided he could not put on his underwear until he had taken his medication! Since he always wore underwear, this pairing worked well for him. For more information on stimulus control procedures, see Martin and Pear (1999).

The clinician should keep in mind that there are actually two things that must be remembered in order to comply with medications: (1) that there is a pill to be taken, and (2) whether or not the pill has been taken. It is common to remember that one is supposed to take a pill, but to forget if one actually took it. Pill dispensers serve as cues or reminders to take medications and also provide a check if the medications actually were taken. There are many different forms of pill dispensers available at local drug stores. Some have dividers for different times of day. Some have a separate section for each day of the week. Some have both features. The child or parent can fill all the relevant sections of the container at a standard time each week (e.g., immediately after getting up on Sunday morning). For the rest of the week, if a pill is in the container, it serves as a prompt to take the medication. If the container is empty, the pill has been taken. This system can be very effective (except when the pill container is accidentally put in the bathroom drawer and forgotten). A chart also can be used to prompt and record when medication has been taken. (See Figure 11.1)

In some cases, it may be necessary to change the person who is responsible for remembering to take the medications. For example, Sue, a very bright, articulate 9-year-old girl, was not taking her scheduled pain medications. Sue was a good student and regularly received commendations from teachers for her conduct at school. But, she was very immature in her assumption of responsibilities at home. She did not pick up her toys, help set the table, or do any other age-appropriate chores around the house. Her mother worked the night shift and a teenage babysitter watched the children in the evenings. In the mornings, Sue's mother was exhausted and went to sleep soon after the children went to school. Sometimes, she worked late and did not arrive home until after the children had left for school.

The evaluation revealed that the mother regularly gave Sue her pain medications with an after-school snack. She expected Sue to remember to take the medications before going to bed and when she awoke. However, Sue rarely

Write the time each day that your child takes his pain medication.
Week of _____

	Sunday	Monday	Tuesday	Wednesday	Thursday	Friday	Saturday
Morning	time:	time:	time:	time:	time:	time:	time:
Lunch	time:	time:	time:	time:	time:	time:	time:
Dinner	time:	time:	time:	time:	time:	time:	time:
Bedtime	time:	time:	time:	time:	time:	time:	time:

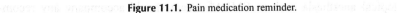

Figure 11.1. Pain medication reminder.

remembered to take the morning and evening doses, and thus received only one dose per day.

The intervention in this case involved shifting the responsibility for remembering the medications to other more responsible individuals in her environment. The babysitter was instructed to administer the nighttime dose immediately prior to putting Sue in bed. In consultation with her physician, the morning dose was rescheduled slightly to allow the school nurse to give her the medication immediately upon arrival at school. (Home health nurses also can supervise medication administration, although it is probably not practical to have a nurse visit several times a day.) By enlisting responsible adults in Sue's environment to help prompt her to take her medications, she was able to improve her medication compliance to acceptable levels.

Provide a More Palatable Form of Medication

Compliance with oral medications sometimes can be enhanced if the medication itself is made less aversive. If pills have an unpleasant taste, they can be crushed and then mixed with another substance to mask the taste. Although the effectiveness of the substance will depend on the taste of the medication and the taste preferences of the child, commonly used agents include applesauce, chocolate ice cream, chocolate milk (Be sure the medication can be paired with dairy products!), or pharmaceutical preparations, such as Syrpulta® (a strongly grape-flavored liquid). Some medications also come in liquid form, making them easier to swallow than a pill. Another advantage of liquid medications is that they can be placed directly into the child's mouth with a syringe, which is often the quickest and most straightforward way to give medication to a toddler. Check with a pharmacy, the nursing department of a children's hospital, or a pediatrician's office for other recommendations. For example, a creative pharmacist offered to crush an unpleasant tasting tablet and fit it into a capsule, so that a child who had trouble swallowing tablets could successfully take the bitter medication without experiencing a gag-inducing unpleasant taste. If the child does not know how to swallow pills or is gagging in the process, the best treatment recommendations may be to change to liquid medication (if the child is under the age of 6) or to teach the child how to swallow pills if the child is older. (See Blount, Dahlquist, Baer, & Wouri [1984], or Funk, Mullins & Olson [1984], for examples of pill-swallowing training programs.)

Protesting when having to swallow a pill and failing to ingest all of the prescribed medication are common in preschool-age children. If possible, a liquid form of medication given via syringe in a very quick, matter-of-fact manner is recommended. However, if cooperative medication ingestion cannot be attained, intravenous or injected forms of pain medication may be needed. A recommendation for topical anesthesia such as EMLA® cream should accompany any recommended invasive medication administration, to prevent unnecessary pain and trauma.

Address Misconceptions and Fears

Some fears that are grounded in misinformation can be eliminated simply through education. For example, many parents and children are reassured and more willing to use the prescribed analgesics when told that the children will not become "addicts" if they take narcotic pain medications. Such reassurance should include explanations of tolerance and addiction at levels appropriate for the educational and developmental level of the child and family. For individuals who believe that it is preferable to tolerate pain as long as possible before "giving in" and taking pain medication, it may be helpful to explain that taking medications when pain is relatively mild (rather than unbearable) may result in the child needing less medication overall (McGrath, 1990). However, if the family's beliefs are incompatible with using a particular type of pain medication, alternative methods of pain control (i.e., non-narcotic medications or nonpharmacological pain control strategies) should be explored.

As is the case with any medication, one must weigh the benefits of the drug against any unwanted side effects. Families that have had bad experiences with drug side effects may be very reluctant to try a pain medication. These concerns are legitimate, but may not have been shared with the physician. Often there is no clear "correct" course of action for the child. Some families and children may choose to experience a greater level of discomfort in order to be able to go to school and function on a day-to-day basis. The clinician, in these situations, often must help family members communicate their concerns to the physician and help both parties reach an acceptable compromise. One patient refused to take his pain medications because they made him nauseous. However, after discussing his concerns, his physician changed his administration schedule so that the medications were taken on a full stomach, and he no longer experienced significant nausea. In contrast, another youngster decided he did not want to receive conscious sedation before painful bone marrow aspirations, because he did not like the "weird" way it made him feel. He opted to experience more pain in order to avoid the disturbing sensations associated with the drugs.

Make Sure Medications Are Available

Often the families that have trouble purchasing medications are not the poorest families. The poorest families may have medical assistance and may have less difficulty obtaining medication than the uninsured "working poor" or middle-class families with mediocre insurance reimbursement. Acknowledging up front that medications are likely to be expensive and providing unsolicited information about sources of financial assistance for medication costs can help families with-

out requiring them to experience the embarrassment of confessing to financial difficulties. Sometimes a simple request for generic forms of drugs can cut families'
costs immensely.

PROBLEM: OTHER PHYSICAL FACTORS ARE EXACERBATING THE CHILD'S PAIN

Help the Child Avoid Protective Posturing

In some cases, providing adequate pain medication may solve the problem of protective posturing. Children assume a protective position to avoid moving in a way
that hurts. If they have adequate pain relief, they can be freer to move about. The
cramped sore neck muscles from holding their bodies in an unnatural position can
then relax and become more comfortable.

At the simplest level, the child should be encouraged to engage in physical
activities deemed safe by the physician. This may require establishing a walking
schedule or periods of time out of bed. For example, we developed a program for a
6-year-old girl recovering from surgery that required her to walk from her hospital
room to the door of the next room, then from her door to two doors down, etc., at
scheduled times throughout the day. In return, she earned TV time or play time
with her mother.

However, if the protective posturing has continued for some time, referral to
a physical therapist may be necessary. The child may need special exercises to treat
muscle atrophy, contractures, and/or other physical complications that result from
extended periods of inactivity or unnatural physical positions or movement.

Improve the Child's Sleep Patterns

One of the quickest ways to improve sleep is to help the child get on a sleep–awake
schedule that parallels "normal" daily activities. If the child stays up very late and
then naps on and off throughout the day, the therapist can begin by eliminating
naps (in older children) or by shortening the amount of time spent napping. The
clinician should keep in mind that one cannot *force* a child go to sleep, but one *can*
keep a child awake. So, the control of sleep is best accomplished by controlling
awake time. If the child spends a developmentally appropriate amount of time
sleeping, but the time of day he/she sleeps is disrupted, and the child is sleeping
during the day and awake at night, a gradual program of progressively later bed-
times (with no napping in between) can be implemented. For example, consider
the 9-year-old child who sleeps from 6:00 A.M. to 4:00 P.M. The total amount of
sleep is appropriate for the child's age (Ferber, 1985), but the timing needs adjustment. According to Ferber (1985) a program for this child may consist of the following:

Day 1	Keep the child up until 9:00 A.M., let sleep until 7:00 P.M.
Day 2	Keep the child up until 12:00 noon, let sleep until 11:00 P.M.
Day 3	Keep the child up until 3:00 P.M., let sleep until 1:00 A.M.
Day 4	Keep the child up until 6:00 P.M., let sleep until 4:00 A.M.
Day 5	Keep the child up until 9:00 P.M., let sleep until 7:00 A.M.

At this point, the child has achieved a more appropriate sleep schedule, which should be followed very consistently to avoid drifting back into the maladaptive pattern. See Weissbluth (1987) and Ferber (1985) for other helpful guidelines for improving children's sleep patterns.

Modify Environmental Variables that Exacerbate Pain

After consulting with school personnel and a physical therapist, if available, any aspect of the environment that unnecessarily exacerbates the child's pain should be modified. For example, an adolescent patient with chronic neck and back pain had to be forced off the couch (where she fell asleep every night watching TV) and into her bed, where the firm mattress could appropriately support her neck and back. Other patients have obtained relief from buying two sets of books—one for home and one for school—to eliminate the strain of carrying them home each day. One teen asked his teachers to keep his textbooks in their classrooms for him, so that he didn't have to carry them from his locker, two stories away. Other aspects of the environment that may help alleviate pain include adjusting seating positions, desk heights, and using ergonomic aids, such as wrist supports for computer keyboards. Physical and occupational therapists can be extremely helpful in identifying the environmental factors that need to be modified and developing the appropriate modifications for the individual child.

Schedule Physical Activities Appropriately

The assessment should reveal the times and types of activity scheduling that are problematic. If inadequate warm-up or comfort measures are used prior to physical activities, the child should be given clear instructions for the appropriate steps to be taken prior to physical activity. For example, everyone should do stretches and general warm-up exercises prior to strenuous exercise. Children with chronic painful conditions may need to use additional comfort measures before even mundane activities. For example, one patient needed to soak in a hot bath in the morning as soon as he awoke in order to be able to dress himself and walk to the bus stop with minimal discomfort. In general, physical activities should be scheduled when the child is most likely to be comfortable and successful in the activity, rather than at times when pain is likely to occur.

Rest periods should be scheduled to *prevent* over-exertion, not to *recover from* over-exertion. Appropriate rest periods can prevent overuse injuries. They also allow the child to direct attention to body cues of fatigue or strain that are likely to be ignored in the midst of activity. This will heighten the child's sensitivity to indications that it's time to stop the activity entirely. Parents and children will need assistance in establishing guidelines for reasonable rest/play time periods. In addition, some sort of incentive system may be needed to ensure the child's cooperation with the rest periods. For example, if the sport is one the child enjoys, daily participation could be made contingent on appropriate warm-up and rest periods the previous day.

Treating Cognitive and Emotional Contributors to the Child's Pain

Developmental issues are of essential importance in designing appropriate interventions to divert the child's attention from the pain stimuli. First, the nature of the diverting cognitive activity must be developmentally appropriate. The child must have the skills to perform the task, and, perhaps even more importantly, must find the task interesting and enjoyable. This requirement eliminates activities like subtracting serial 7s from 10,000 for most children (and most adults). The task would be too difficult for some, and too boring for most children. The two cognitive strategies that are most effective in clinical practice are *distraction* and *imagery*.

Provide Distraction

If the mechanism by which distraction works is, as theory speculates, one of "using up" the child's available attentional capacity (McCaul & Malott, 1984), then the most effective distractor will be the one that requires the largest amount of the child's attention. If the child can easily pay attention to the pain stimulus while engaged in the "distracting" activity, then the distractor is not serving its function. Moreover, if the child tires of the activity, and stops doing it, it will be of little help. Distracting activities can be conceptualized along the following dimensions; maximizing each dimension will make the distractor optimally effective.

Active versus Passive

A passive activity that requires little response on the part of the child is likely to be less effective as a distractor than an activity that requires the child's active participation. Thus, reading a story to a child is better than providing no activity, but will be less effective than reading to the child and asking the child to point to parts of the picture related to the story, or having the child read out loud. The more active the distracting activity, the better. A distractor that requires the child to respond physically or to solve a problem is better than one requiring a simple cognitive or verbal response.

Number of Sensory or Response Modalities Involved

Multi-sensory stimuli tie up more of the child's attention than single modality stimuli. Reading aloud while showing the child pictures is likely to be more effective than simply reading. A movie will be more engaging than an audiotape. Puppet or doll play may add tactile and kinesthetic sensations to verbal and visual stimuli.

Variability of the Distracting Stimuli

In order for a distractor to remain effective it must continue to engage the child's attention. This means the child should not habituate to the stimulus and come to ignore it. The ticking of a new clock might keep someone awake at night for a few days, but it will eventually fade out of consciousness, facilitated by the sameness of the repeated stimulus. Since we do *not* want the child to stop noticing the distractor, it should be variable enough to continue to surprise or otherwise engage the child's attention. Video games are good examples of highly variable stimuli capable of sustaining a youngster's attention for many more hours than most parents would like.

Developmental Considerations

A distractor must also fit the abilities and interests of the child. A 6-year-old girl may find variations on Barbie® doll play optimally distracting. A 9-year-old boy may prefer the latest combat computer game. The toddler may be delighted by pressing the same four buttons over and over to hear a voice say, "Find the cow. The cow says, 'Moo!'" while his teenage sister may prefer to watch a comedy film.

Pilot testing the distractor during non-pain periods will help ensure that it is engaging and appropriate for the child. We have had good success with relatively inexpensive ($25 to $30 range) electronic games available in toy stores, especially those that include different activity cards. The different cards allow one to vary the distractor each time it is used and also often allow for different levels of abilities. For example, one card might require the child to match objects of the same color while another might require the child to identify missing letters in words. Games that have interesting visual stimuli, make sounds, require the child to make a response, and then give feedback have proved to be very effective in our research with children between the ages of 3 and 6 undergoing repeated injections (Gelfand, Pringle, Hilley, Senuta, & Dahlquist, 1998; Landthrip, Pendley,

Dahlquist, & Jones, 1994). For 2-year-olds and young 3-year-olds, simpler electronic toys that make an animal noise, say a sentence, or play a short tune when the child touches the picture work fairly well. Of course, the ability of the distractor to maintain the child's attention will be limited by the attentional capacity of the child. One should not expect hours of uninterrupted play with any activity from a young child.

Older adolescents may be able to use more purely cognitive activities as distractors, in much the same way adults can. Turk, Meichenbaum, and Genest (1983) recommend the following strategies:

> ...counting floor or ceiling tiles, examining the construction of a piece of furniture in the room, carefully examining a garment you are wearing, reading a book, watching television and keeping track of some aspect of the program (p. 291)

With older children, we have used reading aloud, counting the number of polka dots or stripes on the nurse's shirt, and counting the number of times a television character's name is said as distractors.

Practical Considerations

Even the most amusing activity can become tiresome if over-used. Therefore, a variety of distracting activities should be available. Access to the distractors should be limited to the pain periods and not provided routinely throughout the day. This is essential for pain during medical procedures, when the novelty of the distractor helps focus the child's attention away from needles and other frightening stimuli. In chronic pain situations, "real life" often can be the distractor. The more the child engages in normal daily activities, the more likely attention will be diverted away from his/her pain.

Longitudinal group studies of children's responses to distraction interventions are lacking (Dahlquist, 1992). There are some reports of successful use of distraction for up to three consecutive medical procedures (e.g., Landthrip et al., 1994) and encouraging data from a study of four children at 1- and 6-month follow-ups (Powers, Blount, Bachanas, Cotter, & Swan, 1993). We currently are studying the long-term maintenance of distraction effects in preschoolers (Gelfand, Pringle, et al., 1998), but we have not yet completed our long-term follow-up data collection. Until more research is available, clinicians should be careful *not* to assume that children will be able to use the same distraction strategy indefinitely. For example, if the child has a traumatic pain experience, the child's distress may escalate and the child may even refuse to use the distractor entirely. One may need to introduce stricter contingencies at such times, in order to increase the incentives for using the pain management strategy.

This was strikingly illustrated by one 3-year-old patient who was terrified of the intramuscular injections involved in his chemotherapy. Distraction was very effective in reducing his distress to the point that he spontaneously commented, "I'm not even afraid any more!" However, an infection required him to be hospitalized for intravenous (IV) antibiotics. Unfortunately, his veins were very difficult to access, and the medical staff did not use EMLA® cream during their repeated efforts to start his IV line. Not surprisingly, these experiences were extremely painful and upsetting for this youngster. After discharge, his distress during subsequent intramuscular injections returned to baseline levels, requiring re-institution of more intensive interventions to again achieve distress reductions.

Use Imagery

The goal of imagery is the same as the goal of distraction—to divert the child's attention away from the pain experience or the pain stimuli. However, imagery is entirely cognitive in nature, involving no motor activity. The only external stimulus involved is the adult's prompting of the child to imagine a scene that is incompatible with pain or being upset. Turk et al. (1983) recommend the following ways to use imagery to change the pain experience from something noxious to something more tolerable:

1 | *Imaginative inattention.* Imagine doing something that would be incompatible with pain, such as enjoying a fun activity or taking a trip to Disney World.

2 | *Imaginative transformation of the pain sensations.* Imagine that the pain sensations have different sensory qualities that may be easier to tolerate. For example, burning sensations might be imagined as icy cold. Or, the child could imagine his arm is made out of rubber or out of android parts, and therefore can feel pressure, but no pain.

3 | *Imaginative transformation of the pain context.* Imagine the pain occurring in a setting in which it may be easier to tolerate the pain. The child could imagine that she is a superhero injured while making a daring rescue, or a sport star injured during a game who must carry on despite the pain.

Although Turk's imagery work was conducted with adults, there have been several studies applying these techniques with children (e.g., Dahlquist, Gil, Armstrong, Ginsberg, & Jones, 1985; Dahlquist, Pendley, Landthrip, Jones, Wirtz, & Steuber, 1998; Elliott & Olson, 1983; Jay, Elliott, Katz, & Siegel, 1987; Jay, Elliott, Woody, & Siegel, 1991; Gil et al., in press). These techniques are applicable to painful medical procedures, to periods of pain exacerbation following surgery, or to flare-ups of chronic pain conditions, such as Crohn's disease or sickle cell anemia. Clearly, one cannot spend the entire day in fantasy. Imagery, therefore, may be most appropriately viewed as a time-delimited intervention (e.g., to help a child through a 30- to 60-minute medical procedure, or help a child combat exacerbations in pain until pain medications can take effect).

Multisensory Images

The same principles that determine effective distraction should be considered in creating an effective imagery activity. The more interesting and engaging the image, the more likely it will hold the child's attention. Images should be *multisensory* and vivid. "Picture yourself having a nice relaxing day at the beach," is a nice idea, but does not help the child create the image. It leaves the work of the imagery solely up to the child. Few children know how to develop and sustain an image; they need an adult's guidance. After practice, however, older elementary school children may be able to imagine familiar scenes without assistance.

The following is a transcript of imagery instructions for a 10-year-old girl:

> I want you to close your eyes and picture yourself at the beach. It's a perfect beach day. It's warm. The sun is shining, but it's not too hot. You're not even sweating. You're sitting on a brightly colored canvas beach chair. Your feet are in the warm, soft sand. Your eyes are closed. Feel the warm sun on your face. A soft breeze brushes your cheeks and gently blows your hair, tickling your ears for a second. You feel the warmth of the sun on your arms and your legs. The tops of your feet are warm, too. You dig your feet into the sand a little and feel the cool soft sand down deep. Your toes feel a tiny little shell in the sand. As you pick your foot up, the soft sand falls gently over your foot. Your best friend, Amy, is right next to you. She's taking a rest too, since you've both been playing Frisbee. You take a sip of ice cold lemonade and feel the wonderful cool liquid go down your throat. It tastes perfect—just a little tart—not too sweet and not too sour. You lay back with your eyes closed, feeling relaxed and happy. At first all you can hear is the sound of the waves hitting the sand, over and over and over again. You can smell the faint smell of the sunscreen on your arm. As you listen to the waves you start to notice other quieter noises. Seagulls are calling to each other as they dive down to catch fish in the water. There are children playing down on the beach a ways away. You hear their laughter as the waves splash them. Farther down, a dog is trying to catch the waves, barking furiously at each wave he thinks is alive.

This image has many of the qualities of an effective activity distractor. It involves multiple sensory modalities—visual, auditory, gustatory, olfactory, and kinesthetic. It is variable, directing the child to different aspects of the scene over time. It is also developmentally appropriate (assuming the child enjoys the beach).

Tailoring the relaxing image to the individual child can be the most challenging aspect of imagery work. No matter how relaxing the clinician finds sitting in a hot tub or lounging at the pool, if the child isn't interested in the scene, it will become readily apparent. Most children will not keep their eyes closed if they are disinterested in the image.

Whenever possible, the child should be the source of the content of the image. The therapist should ask the child to describe a time he/she felt really peaceful or really happy and then try to get as much sensory detail about the place or event as possible. Since imagery may function not only to divert attention but also to induce relaxation, images that are highly interesting but evoke high arousal or fear should be avoided. Sometimes an unsuitable appearing image can be revised, as in the example of the child who wanted to imagine he was a shark. Although momentarily stumped by her own image of "*Jaws*," the clinician was eventually able to create an image of a benign grandfatherly fantasy shark who cruised the ocean visiting interesting sea creatures. If given a chance, most children over the age of 5 or 6 should be able to participate in generating an image.

If the child is too shy or hesitant to volunteer imagery content, one may want to prepare a few "generic" images likely to be interesting to many children to use in such situations. Sometimes, after a therapist-generated image is used, the child will "critique" the image, suggesting personalized preferences and modifications. Possible images include a magic carpet ride over the child's school or neighborhood, floating on a cloud, playing on the playground, or a visit to the zoo.

One usually can tell by the child's breathing and body posture if he/she is absorbed in the image. The child's eyes should remain closed and his/her body should remain relaxed. If a medical procedure is being conducted, the team members should be informed of the imagery process ahead of time, so that they do not make loud noises or interrupt the child's fantasy with unnecessary questions. One boy was enjoying his imaginary magic carpet ride so much, he invited the physician who was conducting his bone marrow aspiration to join him on the magic carpet. He gave the physician explicit instructions of where he was to sit, to hold on tight, and the good-natured physician agreed to climb on board. The youngster then calmly told the clinician to continue describing his imaginary flight!

It is helpful to make an audiotape of any imagery scenes developed for a child. The child can then draw from a library of tapes to practice in the therapist's absence.

Implementation

Working with the Child

Basic steps in teaching any pain coping strategies are similar to steps that have been found to be effective in teaching any new skill. The clinician should:

1	***Break the task down*** into component steps. Start with easier tasks. Once the child masters the easy steps, more difficult tasks can be attempted.
2	***Explain*** what the child should do and why. Use developmentally appropriate language.
3	***Demonstrate*** what the child should do. Pretend to be the child and role-play using the coping behavior in the pain situation. The child may enjoy pretending to be the parent or teacher or nurse.
4	***Role-play.*** When it is clear that the child understands what is expected, switch roles and have the child practice the coping behavior.
5	***Prompt*** the child to use the coping behavior in the pain situation.
6	***Reward*** the child for successive approximations to the desired pain coping behaviors. For example, preschoolers undergoing injections are asked to play with the distractor at least some time during the injection process in order to receive a small prize. In subsequent sessions, the amount of required interaction with the distractor is increased.

Working with the Parents

Children will not use distraction (or most other pain coping strategies) without the prompting of adults and without some sort of contingencies. We initially discovered this almost by accident. We taught a group of children various strategies to employ during a mildly uncomfortable brief medical procedure, a throat culture (Dahlquist et al., 1986). We made sure each child understood how to perform the coping behavior, practiced it together, and role-played how to use it when they were being examined by the doctor. The actual exam took place a few minutes after our training. However, only about one-third (35%) of the children we trained said they actually did what we taught them to do!

Thus, for most children it is essential that an adult direct the child to use whatever coping strategies are being taught. Until one is certain that the coping strategy will work, this "coach" should be the therapist. This will allow the clinician to fine-tune the coping strategy and solve any unforeseen problems that interfere with its use. Obviously, this is a very time-consuming process and potentially expensive if continued indefinitely. For acute pain related to a medical procedure, it is essential. For more chronic pain conditions, it may be less practical for the clinician to be there whenever the pain surfaces. But, at a minimum, one can try to schedule therapy sessions when the child is actually in pain so that one can coach as well as observe effectiveness first-hand.

Eventually, the goal of treatment will be to turn the "coaching" role over to another adult. Thus, it is crucial to identify someone in the child's environment who can continue to assist the child in the therapist's absence. We use a fading process in which the therapist's involvement gradually diminishes as the parent gradually assumes increasing responsibility for prompting the child to use coping strategies and rewarding the child for doing so (Dahlquist et al., 1998). The therapist demonstrates coaching and gives the parent feedback on his/her performance at each step while gradually turning over responsibility to the parent. Our intervention programs generally follow the following phases:

Phase 1	The therapist prompts the child to use pain management strategies and praises the child's efforts. The parent is instructed to praise the child for following therapist's instructions.
Phase 2	The parent begins prompting the child to use pain management strategies and continues praising child. The therapist also prompts and praises child.
Phase 3	The parent has primary responsibility for prompting and praising the child. The therapist prompts the parent to intervene when needed, gives the parent feedback on his/her performance, but only directly prompts and praises the child if the parent does not respond to the therapist's directions.
Phase 4	The parent conducts all prompting and praising. The therapist observes and gives feedback only.
Phase 5	The therapist is not present. Parents may contact the therapist for phone consultation if needed.

The results of our recent longitudinal study of children undergoing repeated painful chemotherapy procedures strongly support the importance of involving the child's parent in the treatment process (Dahlquist et al., 1998). We compared an intervention program in which therapists provided coaching in pain and anxiety management strategies with a program in which the parents were also taught to serve as their child's coach along the guidelines described above. Although both treatment conditions resulted in clear reductions in the children's levels of distress during the medical procedures, there were two striking advantages to the parent-coaching condition. First, the children whose parents were involved in therapy maintained lower levels of distress after therapy was terminated. Children whose parents participated in coaching also showed reductions in their distress before the painful procedures, whereas the children whose parents were not trained did not improve.

These results confirm the important role that parents can play in modulating emotions in children. By helping the parent become more effective in assisting the child during the painful medical procedures, both the child's distress during the painful part of the procedure and the child's anticipatory anxiety appear to decrease. This suggests that important aspects of parent–child communication may be altered by the parent-training intervention. Perhaps parents feel more competent and less anxious, knowing they can help their child. Perhaps they are applying the techniques they learned to other stressful situations and thereby reducing the level of anxiety experienced by the child. Although the precise mechanisms by which parent coaching exerts its influence are not yet clear, the data from our research and the research of others (e.g., Blount et al., 1992; Blount, Powers, Cotter, Swan, & Free, 1994; Dahlquist, 1998; Manne, Redd, Jacobsen, Gorfinkle, Schorr, & Rapkin, 1990; Powers et al., 1993) suggest that the best outcomes will be obtained if parents are incorporated into the treatment program.

Working with the Medical Team

If the medical staff are aware of the pain management program, they can do much to support the parent's and the child's efforts. In acute pain situations, such as painful medical procedures or painful physical therapy exercises, it is essential that staff understand the intervention so that they can help make the environment conducive to using the pain management strategy. For example, the nurse might have to adjust the way in which a shot is given in order for the child to play a video game while receiving the shot. The nurse may have to sit in a different spot or wait a minute or two before beginning in order for the child to engage in the distracting activity.

Staff may need to be less directive and engage in less discussion of extraneous medical issues while the painful part of the procedure is going on, so that the parent is free to direct all of his or her attention to coaching the child. It may also be necessary to specifically ask that only one person talk at a time, to keep the tension level and noise level in the room under control. Often when a child is highly distressed during a painful procedure, the volume of everyone's voices (not just the crying or screaming child's) escalates as the procedure fails to proceed smoothly. It would be virtually impossible for a child to remain relaxed under such circumstances.

Although we have discussed the feelings of the child and the parent considerably throughout this book, it is important not to overlook the emotions of the health care providers. Many nurses and therapists have revealed personal feelings of failure and/or anxiety when they are unable to effectively help a child manage a painful experience. Their anxiety can make them less competent in a delicate procedure, such as starting an IV in a child's tiny rolling vein. Their anxiety or frustration often is sensed by the child and heightens the child's emotional distress. Thus, it is crucial to present treatment recommendations to medical staff in a way that does not imply they are at fault for the child's difficulties. By giving them an explicit role in assisting the child, one may also help counter any negative reactions that may have developed so far. At the very least, the medical staff should be incorporated into the program at the level of praising the child's efforts to manage the pain.

PROBLEM: ANXIETY IS EXACERBATING THE CHILD'S PAIN

Although distraction and imagery can significantly reduce pain and anxiety, other factors also can contribute to the child's anxiety level and also should be addressed. An overview of the primary strategies recommended for treating cognitive and emotional aspects of children's pain in this chapter are presented in Table 12.1.

Reduce Frightening Aspects of the Environment

Make Sure the Child Has Appropriate Information

In the ideal circumstances, the child will have been provided developmentally appropriate and accurate information about any pain that might occur *prior* to

---

Table 12.1. General Guidelines for Treating Cognitive/Emotional Contributors to the Child's Pain

- Provide distraction
- Use imagery
- Teach coping strategies gradually
  - Break the task down into steps
  - Explain
  - Demonstrate
  - Role play
  - Prompt the child to use the strategy in the pain situtaion
  - Reward coping efforts
- Transfer coaching responsibility to the parents gradually
- Involve the medical team
- Reduce frightening aspects of the environment
  - Provide developmentally appropriate procedural and sensory information
  - Use modeling
  - Minimize separation fears
  - Provide clear signals for the onset and termination of painful events
  - Help adults interact with the child in less frightening ways
- Teach the child anxiety-combating relaxation strategies via demonstration, behavioral rehearsal, *in vivo* practice, and rewards
  - Breathing exercises
  - Progressive muscle relaxation exercises
  - Imagery
  - Positive coping statements
- Provide biofeedback or relaxation training to help reduce physiological reactivity
- Encourage caregivers to address interfering emotional issues in individual or marital/family therapy, or enlist the aid of another adult to assist the child with pain management

its occurrence, whether the pain is the result of surgery, disease process, or a medical procedure. Once a pain problem exists, however, it may be difficult to determine exactly what information the child does or does not have. If the child is facing a relatively new therapy or medical procedure, a developmentally appropriate explanation should be offered. The goal of providing such information is to make any unpleasant or painful aspects of the experience predictable, since predictability facilitates adaptation to aversive stimuli. The literature offers clear guidelines on the most effective ways such information should be delivered.

Provide Procedural as Well as Sensory Information

Providing information about the steps involved in a procedure is important. But it is even more effective if the child also is told what sensations he/she will experience. The now classic study by Johnson, Kirchoff, and Endress (1975) remains one of the best illustrations of this point today. They studied the reactions of children who were having casts removed. All of the children received information about the steps involved in taking off the cast (e.g., First the doctor will saw through the cast. Then the doctor will... etc.). However, some children also were told what they would feel like during the cast removal and the other sensations that they would experience. For instance, they were told how their skin would itch and would look dry and flaky, and they also listened to audiotapes of the sound of the saw used to cut off the cast. They found that the children who received both the procedural and sensory information were much less distressed when their casts were removed than the children who only were told the steps involved in the procedure.

Sensory and procedural information should be conveyed in a developmentally appropriate manner. Thus, for most children, one should demonstrate with objects or dolls, rather than simply explain verbally. Even adolescents and adults benefit from demonstration and diagrams in addition to verbal explanation. There are a variety of puppets and dolls available that can be used to demonstrate surgical techniques or medical procedures. For example, some hospitals use dolls with plastic tubing simulating veins under the doll's "skin." Medical personnel can demonstrate a procedure using the dolls, and children can even practice starting a pretend IV or giving a shot with such dolls in preparation for a novel medical procedure.

If a procedure is going to hurt, it is always better to tell the child ahead of time. Lying to the child is never appropriate. It may work once to "sneak" a painful shot in before the child realizes what is happening. But, it will never work again. The child's trust in what the clinician says will be destroyed. The child may well come to expect pain in many situations that are not actually painful, thus creating a much worse situation.

Use Modeling

Information can also be communicated through peer modeling. Children can learn about a procedure and what is expected of them during the procedure by watching another child go through it. The clinician should keep in mind the factors that have been demonstrated to enhance modeling:

1	The model should be similar to the child (e.g., in age and gender). A 16-year-old boy is not likely to want to imitate a 4-year-old girl!
2	The model should be initially a bit fearful (which makes the model more similar to the child) and then demonstrate appropriate coping with the painful event, rather than being totally fearless right from the start. This coping model (in contrast to the mastery model) allows the child to observe the coping process as well as the successful outcome.
3	The model should be reinforced in some way (e.g., via praise or via a successful outcome of the coping efforts).

However, information in the form of modeling or demonstration primarily addresses anxiety due to missing facts or misconceptions about a painful event. In most cases, this is only one small contributor to the child's overall anxious feelings. For children who have already experienced significant pain, providing such information may be of some benefit, but there are likely to be many more aspects of concern that need attention (Dahlquist, 1992). Thus, informational strategies are probably best employed in a *preventive* fashion. If children are accurately informed *prior* to painful events, they may experience the pain as less noxious and therefore develop fewer negative reactions. (See Dahlquist, 1992, 1997 for additional information on strategies to prepare children for stressful medical procedures.)

Minimize Separation Fears

It is crucial to keep in mind that the concerns of the child may be very different from the concerns of the parents or health care team. Separation often is a major concern, even in older children who have successfully negotiated the transition to the increased autonomy of elementary school. If the child must be separated from his/her parents for medical care, he or she should know where the parents will be and when they will be reunited. If possible, allowing the child to see the waiting room helps make the parents' presence "real." For children with chronic pain conditions, the parents are not likely to be able to be with the child at all times. Thus, it is important to provide a predictable routine that the child can count on. For example, if Johnny knows that Mommy said she will return to the hospital at 5:00, and Mommy always keeps her word, he will not need to worry all afternoon, wondering if something has happened to her. Parental education regarding the importance of structure and predictability should be provided. If the parents are unable to provide this structure and predictability, individual sessions with the parents or family therapy may help identify the psychological or environmental obstacles they are facing.

If parents are unable to spend time with the child, relatives or other adults in the environment may be able to provide some substitute support. For example, a family friend or hospital volunteer may be able to sit with the child for specific, predictable periods of time. Thus, the child can at least count on certain periods of the day during which an adult can advocate for his/her needs. Of course, the parent surrogate also must be reliable.

Provide Clear Signals for the Onset and Termination of Painful Events

It is remarkable how something as simple as signaling the onset of and termination of pain periods can alleviate unnecessary worry about future pain. For example, Derrickson, Neef, and Cataldo (1993) used a light and a buzzer that were turned on at the start of any invasive medical procedure and turned off at the end of the medical procedure for a 9-month-old girl who had lived in the Intensive Care Unit since birth. Prior to using the signal, she consistently showed high levels of negative affect and relatively little positive emotion. However, when provided with the signal—which allowed her to distinguish between "safe" periods versus periods in which uncomfortable procedures would occur, she showed dramatic decreases in negative affect and increases in positive affect as well. Thus, any time a painful or uncomfortable event can be anticipated, it should be accompanied by a clear signal. This is especially important during invasive medical procedures.

Even if the child seems slightly more distressed immediately following the signal, parents and staff should be reassured that some upset is, indeed, appropriate. It is the upset that precedes and follows the painful event that may be unnecessary. Indeed, it may be more of a concern if a youngster under the age of 7 or 8 did not show at least some anxiety in anticipation of a painful event, whether it involves a grimace, a slight tensing, or mild verbal protest. Older children should be able to inhibit most external displays of distress and may already have developed pain management strategies for inoculations, stitches, or other minor painful events. The young child who shows no escape efforts or no anticipatory reaction should be evaluated closely to see if he/she has experienced repeated physical trauma that may have resulted in a learned helplessness reaction. (See Morse & Kelleher, 1977, and Seligman, Maier, & Solomon, 1971, for more information on the unresponsive, passive behaviors that often follow exposure to repeated unpredictable and uncontrollable aversive stimuli.)

Pain signals should be simple and clearly differentiated from the rest of the environment. This does not mean they have to involve elaborate technology. Simple signals can be used, as long as they are used in exactly the same manner every time, For example:

"Here's the owie."

"A little sting, now."

"One, two, three."

"You will feel some strong pressure now."

The following brief statements can be used to signal when the pain period is over:

"The needle is out now."

"OK, rest."

"Let me stop now for a minute."

"It's all done" frequently is said, but often is too vague to be helpful. The child does not know exactly *what* is all done. Given that the distressing aspects of many medical procedures are not just the painful parts, telling a child one is "all done" when the child still may be experiencing something uncomfortable or frightening way may actually confuse the child.

One can also create a "signal" by performing a procedure in a place that is only used for the medical procedure. For example, taking the child to a treatment room is better than performing unpleasant procedures in the child's hospital room. For procedures conducted at home, the child could sit in a special chair in an infrequently used part of the house.

In chronic pain situations, predictability of the onset and termination of some painful events can be signaled by a clock or a timer. For example, one could set a timer at the start of a painful exercise and tell the child he/she can stop when the time goes off. Or, the clinician could structure sitting time so that the child must sit upright during all of a favorite TV show to signal the start and end of the painful period of physical activity (sitting).

Help Adults in the Environment Interact with the Child in Other Less Frightening Ways

Observation of the child while in pain during the assessment/hypothesis testing phase will reveal ways in which adults interact with the child that may be frightening. Often, adults are unaware of how they respond when the child is distressed. Some parents seem almost angry at the child for crying and try to yell at the child until he/she stops. This strategy rarely works. Others repeat themselves over and over, usually saying the same ineffective command or reassuring phrase, such as: "It's almost over, it's almost over..." or "Relax honey, relax honey." In studies of parent–child interactions during painful medical procedures, adult criticism, vague commands, apology, agitation, and reassuring statements do not appear to be helpful (Blount, Davis, Powers, & Roberts, 1991; Bush & Cockrell, 1987; Dahlquist et al., 1998; Dahlquist, Power, & Carlson, 1995; Dahlquist, Power, Cox

& Fernbach, 1994). In fact, many of these behaviors may actually serve to communicate the parent's or medical staff's anxiety to the child. Even young children are quite adept in sensing emotions in adults in general, and particularly in their own parents (Kopp, 1982). In our current research, we are continuing to examine these subtle indicators of parental emotion and exactly how they relate to children's distress in painful medical settings (Gelfand, Dahlquist, & Hass, 1998; Hilley & Dahlquist, 1998; Switkin & Dahlquist, 1998).

One of the goals of intervention, therefore, should be to decrease the amount of anxiety communicated by the adults interacting with the child. Several strategies are possible. For example, in our current parent training program for painful medical procedures, we videotape parent–child interactions during painful procedures and give parents specific feedback on nonverbal and verbal aspects of their interactions with the child (Gelfand, Pringle, et al., 1998). When reviewing the videotaped session, one parent was shocked to hear her voice get louder and louder as the child's distress escalated. She subsequently was able to modulate her voice tone, regardless of the child's distress level.

Designate a Primary Coach

If several adults are interacting with the child, two primary spokespersons should be appointed. Initially, this should probably be one of the health team members who will tell the child what is happening at all stages of the painful event, and the other should be the psychologist or pain management specialist. (This recommendation assumes that the trained professional will be the best able to stay calm in the situation. However, this "hot seat" can be quite uncomfortable if the clinician has concerns about how a supervisor, colleague, or the family is evaluating his/her performance. It is important for the therapist to keep his/her own anxiety under control as well!). If suggested as a way to create less chaos in the environment, rather than as a critique of anyone's interactions, most parents will welcome this reprieve.

The parents then can be eased back into the pain management role with specific guidelines regarding what to say and how to say it. These new parent behaviors should be rehearsed outside of the stressful situation. Since many parents are embarrassed to role-play at first, the therapist should first demonstrate the parent behaviors and then ask the parent to try them. It's a good idea to acknowledge that most people feel awkward the first few times they do such role-playing.

Parents should be encouraged to identify instances when the child uses the coping behavior that is being taught and praise the child. This is one of the most common behavior management deficits in parents—ignoring the child's coping behaviors. Next, specific prompts and commands can be rehearsed. Whenever possible, these prompts should focus on coping and cooperative behaviors, rather than terminating inappropriate child behaviors. Although we will discuss the concepts of differential reinforcement of pain coping behaviors at length in later chapters, praise examples include: "Take a deep breath, Susie. Good! That was a nice long one!", "You're sitting so nice and still; you're such a big boy!", "You were a good helper today, you kept your arm very still while the nurse put in the IV." Using effective prompts and praise not only functions to help the child learn pain management strategies, but also serves the important function of communicating less adult anxiety to the child.

Help Adults in the Environment Manage Other Aspects of Their Emotional Responses

The specific psychological intervention needed will depend on the emotional issues revealed by the assessment of the family. In the pediatric hospital setting individual or family therapy can help parents work through grief or fears related to the child's illness. Financial stresses, problems at work, family logistics, such as the care of siblings, and marital conflict also are common emotional problems dealt with in family therapy. Although the treatment provided to family members may have nothing to do with pain, the byproduct of successful psychological treatment may be a parent who no longer cries constantly or is no longer too depressed to relate to his/her child.

Improve Communication between Parents and the Child

Families who adapt best to difficult childhood medical conditions, in general, have open and honest patterns of communication (Dahlquist & Taub, 1991). This eliminates the need for the child to guess or fantasize about what is wrong. For example, one boy told his therapist, "The way my Mom was crying, I thought for sure I was going to die. But, she was so upset, I didn't dare ask her." In reality, this youngster had an excellent prognosis. His mother was upset about recently being informed that he would be sterile from his treatments. In the meantime, however, the young boy had been terrified, thinking that every pain he felt signaled his impending death. Therapeutic intervention in such cases involves two components: (1) explaining to parents how lying and saying everything is "fine," when obviously it isn't, serves to heighten fears rather than reassure the child; and (2) providing a safe setting for parents to give honest and developmentally appropriate information. It is ultimately much more comforting to a child to hear, "I'm crying because I am sad that you are sick," than to be told nothing is wrong.

Teach the Child Strategies to Manage Anxiety and Physiological Arousal

Despite the best environmental interventions, children may well have good reasons to be anxious. They may be afraid of upcoming events, afraid to return to school, afraid that the pain may get worse. If the fear and anxiety are exacerbating the child's pain, it can be very helpful to learn a relaxation strategy. Often these relaxation exercises are paired with distraction or other cognitive coping strategies to provide the child a "menu" of coping strategies from which to select. We will review briefly three commonly used relaxation strategies for children: breathing exercises, progressive muscle relaxation training, and biofeedback.

Breathing Exercises

We use the paced breathing procedure developed by Elliott and Olson (1983) for children age 5 years and older. Deep breathing is designed to help the child achieve a state of relaxation by regulating the rate and depth of breathing. However, deep breathing may also serve a distracting role, as it does in natural childbirth techniques, by directing attention away from pain and onto the act of breathing. Deep breathing has the added advantage of being simple to do, requiring no special tools, and being incompatible with distress behaviors, such as crying, which often develop a life of their own and seem to heighten the child's distress.

Since breathing exercises have not been specifically studied with children under the age of 5, it is unclear whether younger children can use them effectively. We have had isolated cases of successful applications with 4-year-olds, but in general, our experience is mixed. Therefore, this strategy should be used very cautiously with younger children.

We begin relaxation training, whether breathing exercises or progressive muscle relaxation exercises, with an explanation of the relationship between tension and increased pain experience. This is particularly important for older children who mistakenly think that a relaxation recommendation means the pain is "all in their head." For pain caused by medical procedures, we will ask the child to tense various muscles and imagine how much harder it would be to get a needle through the hard tense muscle than it would be to push a needle into a nice soft muscle. Even young elementary school children seem to understand the idea that when we relax, our bodies get nice and warm and feel better. When we are tense, our bodies feel worse. We explain that we are going to teach the child how to relax his/her body so that the pain (whatever conditions it involves) will not be so bad (e.g., "so it won't hurt as much when the nurse gives you the shot," "so you can do your physical therapy exercises easier," etc.).

The following is a sample transcript of relaxing breathing instructions for a 6-year-old child:

> One of the best ways to stay relaxed is to breathe nice and slow. Does this look like relaxed breathing? (Demonstrates rapid breathing). No. You're right. Relaxed breathing is much slower, like this. (Demonstrates deep inhalation and slow exhalation).

Imagine you are a bicycle tire being pumped up with air and that there is a tiny hole in the tire. How would air come out of the tire? Like this? (Demonstrates whoosh of air). No. It would take a huge hole to make the air come out like that. A small hole would make a sound like this. (Demonstrates slow expiration with hissing noise.) Now, let's pretend together that we are a bicycle tire being pumped up and then we will let the air out very slowly. Take a deep breath and let it out real slowly like this. (Demonstrates) Now you do it with me. Good job! You let the air out nice and slowly!

The clinician should make sure the child makes a slow hissing noise when exhaling in order to be certain that the exhalation is slow. Practice several times until the child can do it correctly several times in a row.

Once the child has mastered the breathing technique, one can introduce **behavioral rehearsal** (e.g., "practicing how to use breathing when you get your shot"). First, the therapist pretends to be the patient, with the child taking the role of the nurse or physician. The child pretends to conduct the procedure while the therapist demonstrates good coping (e.g., "I'm starting to feel a little nervous now, so I'm going to start my breathing exercises... etc."). Then, they switch roles. The therapist pretends to be the nurse conducting the procedure and prompts the child to do the deep breathing. He/she praises the child and gives corrective feedback as needed.

If the parent is going to be present during the medical procedure, the parent also should participate in the behavioral rehearsal. For example, the clinician could pretend to conduct the procedure while the parent prompts the child to take slow deep breaths and praises the child's performance. The clinician should give the child feedback on his/her performance and also give the parent feedback on his/her prompting and praising of the child.

Implementation: *In Vivo* Coaching

As was recommended in the preceding sections involving distraction, the clinician should accompany the child during the medical procedure and coach the child to use the breathing exercises during the event. Coaching involves two components: prompting the child to do deep breathing and praising the child for doing so. It is helpful to first make sure you have the child's attention by making eye contact with the child or directing the child to look at your face. Prompts should be specific, such as "Take a breath *now*," or "Let me hear the hissing." Praise should specify exactly what the child did that was good, for example, "Nice *slow* breathing," or "I could hear a nice long hiss that time."

The parent's role initially should be one of simply praising the child's efforts, rather than also actively prompting, to keep the number of competing commands to the child to a minimum. The therapist can then gradually transfer the responsibility for coaching to the parent and fade out the therapist's direct communication with the child.

Rewards

Few researchers have been willing to ask children to cope with painful medical procedures without rewarding them for doing so. Therefore, there are no studies comparing pain coping interventions with and without rewards. However, our findings that few children reported using coping strategies they had just been taught (Dahlquist et al., 1986) suggest it is unlikely that children will continue to try to use deep breathing exercises without incentives. We use a grab bag of wrapped trinkets of varying size and value to reward children for trying to use the coping strategy the coach prompted them to use. The criterion for the reward is specified ahead of time (e.g., "To get a prize today, you need to do your deep breathing exercises before the shot and when the needle is going into your leg."). If the child is successful, he/she is allowed to pick a prize. The wrapped prizes should be desirable to the child, but need not all be equally attractive. Adding a few extra special prizes to the bag, however, increases the excitement for some children, just as the unpredictable chance of winning a lottery or the big prize award on a slot machine is appealing to some adults. As is true in any shaping program, initial requirements should be set low enough that the child has a good chance of success (e.g., at least one deep breath on command) and then gradually increased (several deep breaths before and during the painful part of the procedure). Some children will test limits and refuse to breathe as prompted. However, even very young children learn quickly to follow the coach's prompts if the rewards are truly contingent and not given when the child fails to meet criterion. Thus, it is crucial to give the reward only if the child meets the predetermined goal. If the goal is not met, it should be acknowledged in a matter-of-fact manner. "I can't give you the prize this time, but I know you can do better next time." The clinician shoud make sure the parents do not focus on the child's failure to obtain the reward.

Progressive Muscle Relaxation Exercises

Deep breathing can be paired very effectively with training in progressive muscle relaxation to help children reduce anxiety associated with pain situations. Although there are several approaches to teaching children to relax (see, for example, Cautela & Groden, 1978), in our research program and in clinical practice, we usually use a tension-release progressive muscle relaxation exercise in combination with deep breathing. Inhaling is combined with muscle tension; exhaling is combined with muscle relaxation. Thus, in some respects, inhalation serves as a cue to initiate the tension-release cycle. The tension-release procedure is adapted from Bernstein and Borkovec's (1973) progressive muscle relaxation program for adults and is similar to strategies recommended in Meichenbaum and Turk's (1983) pain management program for adults. Because the attention spans of children are so much shorter than those of adults, we begin training with a 7-muscle-group modification of Bernstein and Borkovec's progression, rather than the 16 muscle groups they initially teach to adults.

The first step in teaching relaxation is demonstrating how to tense and relax the various muscle groups. Although the child (and the therapist) may initially feel self-conscious doing the exercises while the other individual watches, it is crucial to demonstrate the tensing of each muscle group and to observe the child tensing each muscle group. The child must be able to correctly tense the muscle group before he/she can move on to learning to relax the muscles. Once the child can reliably tense the muscle group without watching the therapist, one can move on to the tension-release relaxation sequence in which, one by one, all of the muscle groups are tensed and then relaxed.

If feasible, the relaxation instructions should be conducted with the child seated in a chair with his/her arms on the armrests or at his/her side, so that they get used to doing the relaxation exercises in a position that could be used in any setting in which the child is sitting. The following is a transcript (with some added commentary) of a relaxation training session with a 7-year-old child.

Today I am going to teach you some exercises that you can use with your relaxing breathing to get even more relaxed. These exercises will help you notice when parts of your body are tense and will help you make those parts of your body more relaxed.

First, if you need to use the bathroom, you should go now. It's hard to relax if you're feeling like you need to go to the bathroom. (Do not forget this step! It's very uncomfortable to try to relax while holding bladder sphincters.)

Let's start with your right arm. (The clinician may need to help the younger child determine which is his/her right and left. If there is any confusion, use "the hand closest to me" or "the hand closest to the wall" instead.) To tighten the muscles in your right arm, make a fist and tighten all the way up to your shoulder. (The child should keep the arm at his/her side and refrain from lifting it up in the air). Pretend you are showing off your muscle for me. Watch me. OK now you do it. Keep it tight, feel it pull? (Have child hold for about 5–7 seconds). Good. (Feel arm to be sure it's tight.) Don't tighten up so hard that it hurts. Now let go. Let your arm relax totally. Let all the tightness run

out of your arm. Notice how different your arm feels when it is relaxed. (Lift arm to see if it is limp.)

Now, this time when you tighten your arm, take a deep breath like we
practiced last time. When you relax, let the air out slowly. (Demonstrate first, then ask the child to practice with you and praise the child's
efforts.)

The clinician should follow the routine described below for each muscle
group:

1	Demonstrate how to tense and relax, have the child try, give corrective feedback, and praise. Then, repeat the demonstration in combination with deep breathing.
2	Have child try relaxing the muscles in conjunction with deep breathing, provide feedback, and praise.
3	Repeat if necessary.

The following are instructions for each subsequent muscle group. Each
time, the clinician should remind the child to tense only one muscle group at a time
and to keep the rest of the body relaxed. Prompts for breathing should be given as
necessary.

1	*Right arm (already done).* Make fist and "muscle."
2	*Left arm.* Same as right arm.
3	*Face.* This may make you feel silly. That's OK. I feel kind of silly when I do it, too. We're going to scrunch up and tighten our face. Frown and wrinkle your forehead. Scrunch up your eyes. Wrinkle up your nose. Clench your teeth together, pull your lips back, and snarl like a dog. Ugh! That feels real tight. But, it feels nice when it relaxes. Now you do it.
4	*Neck and shoulders.* Pull shoulders up toward ears (or push shoulders back into chair).
5	*Abdomen.* Tighten your belly, like you'd do if someone were going to punch you in the stomach. Make your stomach real hard.
6	*Right leg.* Point your toes toward your nose and lift your leg a couple of inches up. This should pull in your calves and thigh. Can you feel it pulling? Don't pull too hard so it hurts. Stop if your leg cramps.
7	*Left leg.* Same as right.

The next phase of relaxation training involves getting the child into a comfortable position and prompting the child to tense and relax each muscle group in

sequence. Therapists should follow the basic guidelines recommended by Bernstein and Borkovec (1973) for any progressive muscle relaxation-training program. Muscles should be tightened for approximately 5–7 seconds (briefer for feet, to prevent cramping) and then allowed to relax for 30–40 seconds. Each muscle group should be tensed and relaxed twice. At the end of the relaxation sequence, while the child remains relaxed, the therapist goes back over each muscle group, instructing the child to relax it a bit further if any tension remains.

Sessions should be tape-recorded so that the child can practice the relaxation sequence at home and in nonpainful situations. A supply of small, inexpensive tape players and headphones should be available to loan to children who do not own a tape player.

The therapist should use a gentle, relaxing voice, but whispering or an excessively hypnotic voice tone is not recommended. To keep children's attention and heighten the distinction between the muscle-tensing period and the muscle-relaxing period, it may be helpful to exaggerate one's voice, for example, "Notice how your muscle is pulling, how tight and tense it feels!" in a louder, more strident voice, followed by a quieter, gentler, "Now relax....and let all the tightness just ease out of your arm..."

The following is a transcript of a relaxation session with a 9-year-old child.

Get into a comfortable position and close your eyes. Concentrate on the muscles in your right arm. I am going to remind you how to tense each muscle and then I will tell you to start tensing. Tense the muscle when I tell you and then relax when I tell you to. Remember to take a deep breath when you tighten the muscle and let the air out slowly when you relax. Let's practice a deep breath. Let me hear the hissing sound. Good. OK, remember that to tense the muscles in your right arm, you make a fist and show off your muscle. OK, take a deep breath and tense the muscle in your right arm. Pull the muscles tight. Feel it pulling. Notice what it feels like when your arm is tensed. Now relax. Let the air out slowly and let your arm get nice and soft and relaxed. Notice how good it feels when you let your arm relax. Let your arm drop down and sink into the chair. Feel how good it feels to be relaxed. Let all the tightness ease away. Let your arm sink into the chair. Now keep that arm nice and relaxed, and pay attention to your left arm... (The session continues with tensing and relaxing each muscle group two times.)

After the left leg has been tensed and relaxed twice, the therapist can then redirect the child's attention to the various muscle groups and encourage the child to relax each group a bit more. The following excerpt follows the tensing and relaxing of the left leg.

Now, stay nice and relaxed for a few minutes. Think about your arms. If you notice any tightness left in your arms, try to make them as relaxed as you can. Think about your face. If you feel any tightness left in your face, try to relax it away... (The therapist proceeds through each muscle group.)

If the child also is using imagery for pain management, a relaxing image can be incorporated at the end of the relaxation sequence and included in the tape recording.

Now, keep your eyes closed and stay in your nice relaxed position. Imagine you are at the beach (or whatever the child's preferred scene is). (Describe the scene in detail for about 5 minutes.)
  Now, I want you to slowly come back to normal alertness. Keep your eyes closed and shake out your legs. Now move your fingers and your arms. Now open your eyes and sit up.

At the end of the relaxation sequence, it is important to assess how the child felt about the procedure. Some adults find relaxation exercises upsetting. Although children generally do not become more anxious during relaxation training, there may be some unpleasant aspects of the relaxation technique. For example, some children may complain that the chair was uncomfortable or that it was hard to keep their eyes closed (younger children mostly). Others are able to identify specific muscle groups that are difficult for them to tense and relax. This problem can be addressed by adapting the tension exercise until they report they can feel the muscle tension. The neck and shoulders are a common problem muscle group. If the child has a handicapping condition or other physical limitations, it is helpful to consult with a physical therapist to determine appropriate tensing and relaxing strategies. (See also Cautela & Groden, 1978).

Biofeedback

An alternative way to teach children to control their autonomic arousal is to provide biofeedback Although the details of treatment vary depending on the developmental capacities of the child, Allen and Matthews (1998) report that treatment typically involves four clinic visits over an 8-week period in combination with daily home practice. The child is hooked up to a biofeedback apparatus that senses finger temperature or muscle tension. (Temperature is the simplest method to use and is easily transported to a variety of situations.) Each session consists of a period of adaptation to the apparatus, baseline assessment, and then 10–15 minutes in which the child attempts to raise finger temperature (or lower muscle tension).

The biofeedback unit provides immediate information to the child regarding changes in his/her physiological status. The form of the feedback varies, depending on the equipment. Units may display the actual finger temperature via numbers on a dial, may indicate degrees of temperature *change* relative to the baseline temperature, may activate a light that stays on as long as temperature is increasing, or may generate a tone that changes in pitch and frequency as temperature changes (e.g., beeps that become higher pitched and faster as temperature goes down). Some units drive elements of video games, although the research is less extensive with such units. Home temperature training units also are available.

In the first biofeedback session, the therapist may guide the child through images suggesting relaxation or warmth and instruct the child to use these images or develop his/her own imagery to use in practice at home and in subsequent clinic sessions. Since the amount of symptom improvement appears to be strongly related to the amount of home practice (Allen & McKeen, 1991), it is important that children practice daily (Allen & Matthews, 1998).

According to Allen and Matthews (1998), biofeedback tends to be most effective in *preventing* pain episodes, rather than reducing the intensity of pain once it occurs. They argue that "frequent use of biofeedback may reduce reactivity and thereby prevent the onset of painful episodes" (p. 276). Thus, biofeedback may be best suited for recurrent episodic pain problems, such as headaches and recurrent abdominal pain, rather than for acute postoperative or procedural pain, or chronic unremitting pain conditions.

PROBLEM: THE CHILD ENGAGES IN SELF-DEFEATING THINKING ABOUT THE PAIN

Replace Maladaptive Cognitions with Adaptive Cognitions and Coping Statements

Cognitive interventions to combat anxiety-inducing thoughts frequently are used in combination with other relaxation strategies as part of a cognitive–behavioral pain management "package" (e.g., Dahlquist, 1992; Dahlquist et al., 1998; Gil et al., in press; see Table 12.2). Most of these cognitive coping skills training interventions involve the following basic steps:

1	Explain how negative thoughts can make a person feel more worried and feel more pain.
2	Identify worried or negative thoughts the child has had.
3	Identify positive thoughts the child could use to replace these negative thoughts.
4	Demonstrate how the child could use positive coping statements in a painful or stressful situation.

Table 12.2. Replacing Maladaptive Cognitions with Adaptive Cognitions

Negative self-statements	Positive self-statements
I hate this	I can handle this
I can't stand it anymore	It will be over soon
I want my Mommy	If I relax, I will feel better
I'll never get to sleep	I'm strong
This won't help	I'm going to show my mom how good I am at
I'll never get to do anything fun	relaxing
It's not fair	I can manage my pain
Nothing helps, so why should I bother trying?	I've handled pain like this before; I can do it
This is awful	again
I give up	Every time I practice managing my pain, I get a
	little better at it

5	Have the child practice saying positive coping statements to himself/herself.
6	Have the child practice combating negative statements outside of the therapy session.

Gil and colleagues (in press) argued that clinical pain often is unpredictable, uncontrollable, and very intense. Under such circumstances, it may be very difficult for children to concentrate and apply a new skill. Consequently, Gil and colleagues added an additional component to their cognitive coping skills training—the opportunity to practice using positive coping statements while the child is exposed to laboratory-induced pain. The advantage of their approach is that it allows the child to practice with real pain, gives the therapist some control over the intensity of the pain, and allows the therapist to gradually expose the child to increasingly intense pain stimuli as the child practices using coping strategies. Although their approach has not yet been compared with more traditional cognitive strategies, it appears to offer considerable promise.

PROBLEM: THE PAIN HAS SPECIFIC MEANING FOR THE CHILD

Provide Education

If the significance attached to the pain experience is based on misinformation, it may be possible to change the emotional valence of the pain experience relatively easily with accurate information. For example, the child with phantom limb pain who thought his amputated leg was haunting him was immediately relieved when the phenomenon of phantom limb pain was explained to him. Similarly, the child who thinks his pain means he is going to die may be able to view the situation in a much more positive light when assured his condition is not terminal.

Explore Ways to Minimize the Negative Implications of the Pain

For many children, the disability that accompanies a pain problem may be the source of their distress, rather than the actual discomfort. For example, one pain patient was extremely upset by the thought that, because of his illness, he might never play college baseball. After discussing the issue over the course of a few therapy sessions, however, he was able to reconceptualize the situation in a way that helped him feel less hopeless. First, he was able to acknowledge that his chances for a college baseball scholarship might be slim. However, this did not mean he would never be able to play baseball again. The reasons behind his desire to play college baseball were explored. Was it for the love of the game? If so, then how might he continue to play ball even if not on a college team (e.g., through community leagues, coaching Little League, etc.)? If college baseball was important to him because it was his only plan for college funding, then he needed to begin finding alternative ways to fund his education. Once he abandoned the notion that his life was over because of this pain problem, he began working harder on pain management strategies and started trying harder to do well in school.

PROBLEM: THE CAREGIVER'S EMOTIONAL STATUS IS INTERFERING WITH HIS/HER ABILITY TO HELP THE CHILD MANAGE THE PAIN

The many different personal and family issues that might interfere with the caregiver's ability to help the child are far beyond the scope of this book. In some cases, individual or family therapy may be needed in addition to the child's pain management program. However, clinicians should also consider the possibility that another adult may be able to stand in for the parents and assist the child with pain management. In a hospital setting, nurses and child life workers may be able to fulfill this role. In schools, the teacher, school nurse, and counselors may be able to provide assistance.

Treating Behavioral Contributors to the Child's Pain

Once a detailed analysis of the contingencies maintaining the child's pain behaviors and the behaviors of the adults in the environment has been conducted, it should be clear where changes are needed. The same principles underlying good behavior management programs also apply to behavioral interventions for pain. For beginning clinicians, books by Gelfand and Hartman (1984) and Martin and Pear (1999) provide excellent introductions to the processes of behavioral assessment and behavior modification. The recommendations that follow assume that the clinician has some basic experience with behavior management interventions. Hence, the focus is on the unique challenges faced in designing behavior management interventions for pain problems.

PROVIDE A RATIONALE FOR CHANGING EXISTING CONTINGENCIES THAT THE CHILD AND FAMILY CAN UNDERSTAND AND ACCEPT

Just as misconceptions regarding pain and pain medications can influence how families respond to a child's pain, beliefs about treatment can influence their willingness to cooperate with a behavior management plan. Ideally, family concerns about what it might mean to receive psychological help for pain management will have been revealed in the assessment. However, even if families have not specifically voiced any concerns, we find it useful to anticipate that the following concerns are likely to be raised by a friend or family member. Anticipating these concerns will help families see treatment as being compatible with their personal beliefs and values.

As Turk, Meichenbaum, and Genest (1983) point out, most pain patients view their problems "in purely physical terms, rejecting psychological explanations of symptoms. Patients are therefore likely to approach therapy with a view of their problems that does not render them amenable to change...The problem at the outset of therapy, then is to alter the patient's conceptualization so that a psychologically based intervention is feasible. Until some *shared conceptualization* of the therapeutic situation is reached, therapist and patient are likely to be working at cross purposes." (p.154)

The following suggestions are offered as ways to achieve a more shared conceptualization of the child's pain problem.

Use Terminology that Is Not Likely to Offend or Scare Off Family Members

A "reward program" or an "incentive program" may sound less ominous than a "behavior management program" or a "contingency management program." Being referred for "pain management" is more acceptable to many people than being referred for "psychotherapy" or "family therapy."

Clarify that Using a Reward Program in No Way Implies that Anyone Thinks the Child Is Deliberately Faking Pain

The need for extra incentives stems from the fact that learning to control pain is difficult for anyone, and especially hard for children. Therefore, children need recognition and encouragement to keep working at it.

Explain that the Parents Are Not to Blame

Parents often functionally maintain their child's problems. However, if the parents must, in effect, admit to primary responsibility for their child's problems before a treatment program can be initiated, few parents will ever make it to treatment. Fortunately, it is possible to engage parents in a behavior management program and help them change their behavior in many ways without forcing them to "confess" their previous errors. For instance, it is helpful to give parents an "out" or a way to conceptualize their child's problems that saves face and puts the blame on the situation, rather than the individuals involved.

A youngster referred for poor cooperation with injections is a good example. His family saw him as sort of amusingly stubborn and "spoiled" at home, but did not think his behavior was a problem at home or at school. In contrast, the medical staff saw him as extremely noncompliant and a tremendous management problem in the clinic. Based on our observations of this youngster, he appeared much more oppositional than the majority of children his age. We suspected his noncompliance was not unique to the medical situation and would soon become a problem in school and eventually also at home, if his parents began setting more limits. His mother reinforced his negative behavior with attention and provided little reinforcement for compliance or other pain coping behaviors. Since she did not perceive his behavior outside the medical setting as problematic, we did not expect her to be interested in a general parent-training program. However, his behavior during procedures definitely warranted psychological intervention.

Rather than directly confront what appeared to be her poor behavior management skills, we offered her the following rationale:

> Joe is a strong-willed young boy who stands up for himself. As he grows up, this quality will probably be one of his strengths and may help him deal with adversity without giving up, change things that need changing, or may make him an influential leader or a good ball player. However, right now he's directing all his efforts at fighting something that just can't be changed—the fact that he needs to get these painful shots every week. So, what we need to do is help him redirect his fighting spirit in a more helpful direction—toward mastering this difficult situation. Since you are the person who is likely to have the strongest influence on his behavior, you are the best person to help him and provide him incentives for trying to handle these shots. So, what we would like to offer is to work together with you and Joe to find the most effective ways to help him deal with the shots and to build in incentives for him, so that this difficult task feels worth all of his hard work.

For other chronic pain conditions, a modification of Fordyce's (1976) or Turk et al.'s (1983) conceptualizations of chronic pain can be offered to the family to help explain the role of learning in maintaining pain behaviors. For example, the following rationale (modified from Fordyce, 1976) could be offered.

> Imagine you have not eaten all day and you are really hungry. You are walking home from school and your friend starts telling you about the barbecue party he is going to have over the weekend. As he describes the barbecued chicken, done just the way you like it, with lots of sauce, the corn on the cob, and the apple pie, your mouth starts to water in anticipation of the tasty meal.
>
> Your mouth watering is very real. You can feel the saliva. It's not in your imagination. But, there is no actual food around. Your body is reacting to a learning effect that is not under your control. Your body associates thoughts about food with eating and responds as if you were ready to eat. This is a form of automatic learning.
>
> Pain can also become automatically associated with certain things or events. This learned pain is just as real as pain caused directly by an injury. But, the good thing about learned pain is it can be unlearned. That is one of my jobs—to help you unlearn as many of these pain associations as possible.

Table 13.1. General Guidelines for Treating Behavioral Contributors to the Child's Pain

- Provide a rationale for changing existing contingencies that the family can accept
- Define the child's target pain behaviors
- Specify the desired adaptive behaviors to be increased
- Modify contingencies affecting the child's behavior
  - ○ Stop the positive reinforcement of pain behaviors
  - ○ Prevent escape or avoidance via pain behaviors
  - ○ Reinforce adaptive behaviors
  - ○ Prevent punishment of adaptive behaviors
- Provide necessary skill training
- Identify problematic and appropriate adult target behaviors
- Modify contingencies affecting adult behaviors
  - ○ Stop reinforcement of problematic adult behaviors
  - ○ Prevent escape or avoidance
  - ○ Reinforce adaptive adult behaviors
  - ○ Minimize punishment of adaptive adult behaviors
- Provide skills training as needed

Emphasizing how the child's illness or injury "sets up" a situation in which it is almost inevitable that some of these problems develop also may help make the treatment plan seem less threatening to the parents.

If a satisfactory conceptual framework can be offered to the parents, one can then proceed with the actual behavioral intervention. The specific contingency program developed will depend on the results of the previously described hypothesis generation and testing process. In most instances, the final behavioral program will address most of the guidelines presented in Table 13.1 and in the following text, but in an individualized fashion.

DEFINE THE TARGET BEHAVIORS

Clearly Distinguish Problematic Pain Behavior from Legitimate Pain Reports

Because pain serves as an important signal of underlying disease processes in some instances, one cannot simply assume that pain behaviors are always behavioral excesses and therefore should be decreased or eliminated. In fact, ignoring some pain behaviors could actually be harmful for the child. For example, it is appropriate and necessary when drilling a tooth to ask that the child signal if pain is felt, since pain may indicate inadequate anesthesia. Similarly, a physical therapist may suggest that a muscle be stretched to the point where it begins to feel uncomfortable but stretched no further. In such cases, it is important that the child indicate when he/she has pain or discomfort—the pain serves an important signaling function.

Similarly, if a medication is expected to provide 6 hours of pain relief, but the child is feeling pain after about 4 hours, this information should be conveyed to the physician, so that the medication schedule or agents can be adjusted. For certain medical situations, specific pain symptoms are very important diagnostic indicators and should never be ignored. For example, if a child is receiving IV fluids (the needle has already been inserted) and the IV site begins to hurt, this may be an indication that the site has infiltrated (the fluid is no longer just going into the vein, but rather into surrounding tissue). One patient experienced a severe chemical burn on her hand because medical staff ignored her pain complaints as the highly irritating chemotherapy agents infiltrated the tissue in her hand. Other changes in disease status are signaled by changes in pain symptoms (e.g., bone pain may indicate relapsed leukemia, sharp abdominal pain may signal appendicitis) (Kunz & Finkel, 1987). In children with recurrent abdominal pain, when pain is accompanied by certain "red flags," such as "fever, weight loss, blood in the stools, changes in bowel function, pain awakening the child at night, [and] anemia..." it often indicates an organic cause for the pain (Rappaport & Frazer, 1995, p. 278). Such pain symptoms should *not* be targeted for elimination.

The parent or the psychologist should not try to determine which pain symptoms warrant medical attention without consulting the child's physician. The physician should be able to help the pain management professional distinguish dysfunctional pain behaviors from important physiological signals. For example, one child with serious systemic JRA complained daily that her pain was so severe that she could not attend school. Her mother often allowed her to stay home when she complained of pain, because she did not want to be "unfair" and force her to go to school if her disease actually was flaring. By working with her rheumatologist, we were able to develop an operational definition of "clinically significant symptoms" that distinguished signs of disease flare-ups from the chronic pain inherent in arthritis with which the youngster would need to learn to cope. In this child's case, the physician suggested that only if pain were accompanied by fever greater than 101 degrees, could the child stay home from school. At those times, the parent needed to call the physician's office to determine if the child had to be seen.

If one has established clear guidelines regarding the noteworthy pain behaviors that require medical intervention, the parent is likely to be much more comfortable following any subsequent behavioral guidelines that may be recommended. It would do little good to instruct a parent to ignore pain behaviors he or she believed indicated a serious medical problem that warranted immediate attention. Indeed, the mother of one patient reported that she felt as though a burden had been lifted off her shoulders once it was clarified when her daughter should stay home from school. The responsibility of making the decision daily without the necessary medical background had made her very anxious. If she found herself at all uncertain, she tended to err in the direction of giving in to her daughter's requests to stay home, and thereby negatively reinforced many of her pain complaints. Once she had clear guidelines to fall back on, she felt much more confident about enforcing school attendance. In this family, the parent's concerns and beliefs were inextricably tied to her willingness and ability to follow through with any behavioral recommendations.

Specify the Desired Behaviors that Need to Be Increased

If the child were appropriately handling his/her pain, what behaviors would be expected? In other words, how will all parties involved know if the child is doing a good job? What are the ultimate goals for this child? It is important to clarify the positive target behaviors as well as the negative targets before proceeding with a behavioral intervention.

The desired behaviors must be developmentally appropriate and also reasonable in light of the child's medical status. Consider for example, the father who wanted his 5-year-old son to go through an unsedated lumbar puncture without crying. When we started working together, the frightened boy was crying from the moment he heard he was going to get the procedure until it was over and he returned to his room. His father continuously berated him for crying. The first step in intervention, then, was to help his father set a more realistic goal for his son. Crying when something hurts is developmentally appropriate for a 5-year-old child. Telling a child he may not cry is unreasonable and possibly harmful, if the child is made to feel like a failure in his unsuccessful attempts to achieve this unrealistic goal. However, screaming and kicking long before the procedure starts is not the highest level of emotional control one could expect of a 5-year-old. Given that this child exhibited extremely high levels of distress, we recommended the following initial target behaviors:

1 | Allowing the nurse to move him into position;
2 | Holding still while the doctor did the lumbar puncture; and
3 | Doing breathing exercises on command.

Crying was not targeted at all. With intervention, the youngster was able to achieve these goals and earn his father's praise rather than disapproval. Although not directly targeted, his crying in anticipation of the pain of the procedure also decreased.

The specific positive behaviors selected will depend on the child's age and circumstances. Possible target behaviors may include attending school, getting out of bed, sitting in a chair, doing exercises, walking without assistance, using a pleasant voice tone, practicing relaxation, and playing with a distractor. The key is making sure that the parent, child, and health professionals involved all understand the goals for the child, so that inconsistencies or conflicting messages to the child are avoided.

PROBLEM: THE CHILD'S PAIN BEHAVIORS
ARE POSITIVELY REINFORCED

Remove the Reinforcement for the Pain Behaviors
and Reinforce Adaptive Behaviors

Although this may seem relatively straightforward, this may well be the most difficult thing for most parents and caregivers to actually do. Cries of pain have tremendous power to elicit responses from adults. Many parents report that their child's pediatrician told them there was nothing seriously wrong with their child and that they should "just ignore" their child's pain complaints. However, they complained that this was "impossible" and, furthermore, that the pediatrician just didn't understand how badly their child was hurting.

Extinction strategies such as ignoring should never be the only behavioral intervention used. Extinction should only be used in conjunction with rewarding a replacement for the pain behavior.

With this caveat in mind, there are a variety of ways to help parents and/or medical staff stop providing positive consequences for pain behaviors and begin rewarding desired behaviors. Gifts and toys and special treats for the sick child can be held in reserve for days the child does an especially good job of managing his/her pain. For example, the special gift from Grandma could be opened the day he went to school despite pain, rather than the day he stayed home because he had too much pain to go to school.

If the child's pain behaviors appear to be reinforced by adult attention, one can teach the adults to use differential attention to reinforce behaviors that are incompatible with pain complaints. Consider again the example of the 4-year-old girl recovering from surgery that was presented in Chapter 10. Evaluation revealed that her mother talked to her and otherwise attended to her whenever she whimpered, but when she was silent, her mother resumed reading her novel. During treatment, we taught her mother to ignore the child's whimpers by picking up her novel and starting to read, and to respond with verbal attention whenever her daughter was not whimpering. We employed the differential attention strategies outlined in Forehand and McMahon (1981), which simply involve providing an ongoing verbal commentary on the child's behavior as long as the child is behaving appropriately and ignoring inappropriate behavior. It is remarkable how powerful such a simple intervention can be. Children seem to relish the undivided attention of an adult and quickly determine the behaviors to which the adult is responding.

However, the corresponding ignoring of unwanted pain behaviors can be very difficult for adults. Often they will provide elaborate explanations of how they are going to ignore the child, all the while attending to the very behaviors they purportedly plan to ignore. Therefore, it is important to specify precisely *how* the adult should ignore the pain behaviors. What should the adult do while ignoring? Should he/she look away, turn around, leave the room, talk to someone else? At the very least, the adult should not speak to the child and should probably turn away or avert his/her gaze.

Sometimes it is impossible not to attend to pain behaviors unless one leaves the room. In this fashion, the parents create a time out from reinforcement by removing themselves (the source of social reinforcement) from the child. As is the case any time extinction is used, parents and staff should be prepared for an escalation in pain behaviors (an extinction burst) before the pain behaviors diminish. For example, the child may cry louder and complain more vehemently in order to try to regain the adult's attention.

PROBLEM: THE CHILD'S PAIN BEHAVIOR IS NEGATIVELY REINFORCED

Prevent Escape or Avoidance and Reinforce Adaptive Behaviors

Regardless of the nature of the aversive stimulus, as long as the child's pain behaviors are effective in avoiding or escaping it, the pain behaviors are not likely to diminish. This is most obvious when pain allows the child to avoid going to school or escape an unpleasant class or activity. Treatment should focus on requiring the child to remain in school or remain in class despite the pain. It may be necessary to shape successive approximations of the adaptive behavior (e.g., school attendance) that will eventually replace avoidance.

The following shaping program was used with one patient for whom school avoidance negatively reinforced pain complaints. In order to earn access to daily and weekend privileges, he was required to stay in school all day.

Week 1	He had to remain in the school building, rather than go home. He could lie down for as long as he desired in the nurse's office if necessary.
Week 2	He could request pain medication from the nurse, but had to sit up and work on schoolwork in the nurse's office.
Week 3	He could request pain medication from the nurse, but only at specified time periods, and had to return to class after about 10

	minutes. Teachers were instructed to ignore pain behaviors in class, such as resting his head on his desk, etc.
Week 4	Contingencies from week 3 remained in effect. However, natural consequences began to exert some control over his behavior. He spontaneously stopped putting his head down on his desk out of embarrassment and became more active in trying to use distraction and other pain management activities without leaving the classroom.

Caution: Be Consistent

The key to successful treatment in any behavioral intervention is consistency. Once a decision is made to keep the child in school despite pain, it must be enforced for every pain episode. If not, the pain behaviors will be intermittently reinforced and even harder to change in the future.

However, remaining steadfast in resolve is more difficult when the child is complaining of pain than when the child is behaving in a more obviously inappropriate manner (e.g., throwing a temper tantrum). Thus, it is crucial that all parties involved in enforcing the termination of negative reinforcement of pain behaviors are in agreement. Having a predefined, clear idea of pain behaviors that do and do not warrant medical attention will help all parties remain consistent.

Continue to Reinforce Adaptive Behavior

It also is crucial that the child's pain coping efforts be positively reinforced. Once a child begins to show less pain, it is easy for those around him/her to take this improved behavior for granted and no longer positively reinforce it. Initially, every instance of adaptive behavior should be positively reinforced. Later, the schedule of reinforcement can be faded to a more intermittent schedule. For example, one could begin with hourly stickers for appropriate self-help behaviors and then fade to praising self-help behaviors at random times throughout pre-specified time periods during the day. (For more information regarding schedules of reinforcement and fading procedures, see Martin & Pear, 1999.)

PROBLEM: THE CHILD'S ADAPTIVE BEHAVIOR IS PUNISHED OR INADEQUATELY REINFORCED

Prevent/Remove the Punishment

This may be one of the most challenging aspects of pain management for chronically ill children. Returning to normal daily activities is hoped to increase the child's access to a variety of positive stimuli that will help maintain the adaptive behaviors. However, some children continue to experience extremely aversive consequences when they begin to function more appropriately.

For example, the child may return to school only to face ridicule and teasing from peers. Efforts should be made to anticipate possible negative consequences of returning to school. Peer teasing can sometimes be prevented if a teacher discusses the child's illness with the class before the child returns to school. This can be particularly helpful for children experiencing dramatic changes in their appearance, such as hair loss from chemotherapy or significant weight gain from corticosteroids. Older children may benefit from a "buddy" arrangement, in which a competent peer accompanies them from class to class, helping them find their classroom, getting make-up assignments, and assisting in defending against any peer ridicule.

Behaviors that are certain to result in negative consequences should not be recommended. For example, a child should not be encouraged to engage in a sports activity without adequate practice and preparation. Remediating skill deficits also will help prevent punishment of the child's efforts to behave adaptively.

Reinforce Adaptive Behavior

Mild punishment is inherent in some adaptive behaviors. For example, physical therapy and other forms of rehabilitation may be uncomfortable, inconvenient, and time-consuming. Any one of these factors could punish the child's behavior. Similarly, getting up early in the morning, doing one's homework, or getting dressed without assistance take more effort than the more maladaptive behaviors of lying in bed, doing nothing, being waited on, or being helped with dressing. Thus, considerable reinforcement will be needed in order to overcome these punishment contingencies.

Even if the punishment of adaptive behavior can be prevented, there is still a need to reinforce the child's adaptive behaviors. Simply removing the punishment does not necessarily insure that the child will behave adaptively. Immediate reinforcers should be provided for the adaptive behaviors desired for the individual child. As discussed previously, the positive goals for the child should be defined idiographically. The same goals may not be appropriate for different children.

PROBLEM: THE CHILD LACKS SKILLS NECESSARY TO PERFORM ADAPTIVE BEHAVIORS

Provide Skill Training

The child may need focused education in specific skills before he/she can actually perform the adaptive behaviors that are desired to replace the pain behaviors. Some examples of skills that may be deficient are presented in Table 13.2.

Table 13.2. Potential Skill Deficits

1. Peer initiation skills
2. Conflict resolution skills
3. Study skills
4. Note-taking skills
5. Emotion identification/communication skills
6. Information-processing skills
7. Problem-solving skills
8. Cognitive distraction skills
9. Progressive muscle relaxation skills
10. Imagery skills

CASE EXAMPLE

Jessica, a 12-year-old girl with fibromyalgia was referred for pain management. Although she professed a strong desire to get better and return to school, she was very noncompliant with self-monitoring requests. She claimed she forgot to bring in her rating sheets three sessions in a row. In the meantime, she continued to miss 3 to 4 days of school per week because of pain. Her frustrated therapist determined that he was not likely to get compliance with self-monitoring. So, he switched the focus of treatment from her subjective experience of pain to the permanent product of her pain behaviors, school attendance. In cooperation with her mother, a behavioral program was established in which avoidance of school because of pain was no longer allowed, and positive consequences were established for school attendance. If Jessica felt pain in school, she was instructed to redirect her attention to the teacher or to school assignments. She was not allowed to stay home from school or come home early if she felt pain. All social and leisure activities were made contingent upon school attendance. Jessica could earn the privileges of shopping, dances, and movies. if she attended school every day.

Jessica's mother accepted these contingencies as extreme measures needed to motivate Jessica to learn to handle her potentially lifelong pain condition. She enforced the behavioral program consistently. Jessica was furious at the therapist, but she responded very well to the contingencies. She attended school every day and ultimately successfully completed middle school and high school.

WORKING WITH THE PARENT AND THE HEALTH CARE SYSTEM

Identify Problematic and Appropriate Adult Target Behaviors

In most cases, in order for a child's pain problem to resolve, both the child's behavior and the behavior of the child's family members and any other individuals car-

Table 13.3. Operational Definitions of Problematic and Appropriate Parental Behaviors

Problematic parental behaviors	Appropriate parental behaviors
• Attends to child pain behaviors	• Ignores all but medically significant pain behaviors
• Negatively reinforces child pain behaviors (i.e., allows child to avoid school because of pain)	• Reinforces child for attending school despite pain
• Fails to give appropriate around-the-clock medications	• Administers medications on around-the-clock schedule as prescribed
• Ignores child when pain-free	• Praises child's independent pain management efforts

ing for the child may need to change. For simplicity, we will discuss parent behaviors in the following sections. However, the same principles could apply to the behavior of nurses, teachers, rehabilitation therapists, and others.

In order to know where to begin to intervene, it is helpful to conceptualize maladaptive parental behaviors in much the same fashion as we have conceptualized the child's maladaptive pain behaviors. In other words, the clinician should develop an operational definition of the parental behaviors that are not helping the child and then identify the parental behaviors that would be more helpful for this child. Table 13.3 lists several common problematic parental behaviors and the more appropriate behaviors one would hope to instill in their place.

PROBLEM: THE ADULT'S PROBLEMATIC BEHAVIOR IS POSITIVELY REINFORCED

Remove the Reinforcement for the Adult's Problematic Behavior and Reinforce Appropriate Adult Behaviors

If the adult's responses to the child's pain appear to be maintained by the positive interactions with the child that follow, it is important to help the parent find other ways to nurture the child and achieve closeness without attending to pain behaviors. For example, one could schedule special times for cuddling and sitting close together that are likely to be enjoyable for both the child and parent, but do not depend on the child being in pain in order to occur. A bedtime routine involving story time or talking together about the child's day (for older children) may provide the intimacy and closeness the parent enjoys, without the risk of inadvertently reinforcing the child's pain behaviors.

In a broader systemic sense, the health care team also may need to change how they respond to parental reports of the child's pain. If the physician orders extensive tests every time the parent reports pain symptoms, there is no way the parent is going to stop attending to the child's pain! At some point the health care provider must stop reinforcing the parental attention to the child's pain by declining to conduct further tests. Otherwise, the message communicated to the parent is, "yes, this pain is serious and may warrant medical attention." One cannot give this message and also expect a parent to ignore pain reports.

For parents who enjoy the support and attention from the medical staff, it is important not to cut them off from this attention when the child improves. The psychologist ultimately may need to work with the parents to develop alternative sources of social support and attention. In the meantime, the medical staff can redirect their support to the parent's efforts to help the child cope with the pain, return to school, etc.

The mother of a 6-year-old cancer survivor illustrated this issue very well. For two years, her daughter's medical care had required frequent hospitalizations and at least once-a-week visits to the medical center. Her mother had to quit her job in order to take her child in for medical care. As a result, her social contacts were restricted to the parents of other ill children and to the medical staff providing her daughter's care. Her marriage was unhappy and conflicted, which further restricted her sources of support outside the medical setting.

Her daughter completed treatment and was in complete remission. Her immune status was excellent, and she was ready to return to school. However, her mother seemed unduly concerned about minor aches and pains and repeatedly kept her home from school and brought her to the clinic for these unimportant pain complaints. Her inappropriate attention to her daughter's symptoms and her failure to encourage her daughter to go to school was reinforced by the attention and support from the medical staff she received each time she brought her daughter in for an appointment.

We attempted to address this problem by scheduling "well child" check-ups at much more frequent intervals than would normally be required so that she could obtain support and attention from the medical staff without her daughter having symptoms. We also arranged for one of the staff nurses to call her at home daily and praise her efforts to get her child back in school. Finally, we provided individual therapy to directly address her needs for attention and support, so that there would be less need for her daughter to be ill in order for the mother to have someone with whom she could talk. Over the course of therapy, the frequency of medical staff contacts was gradually faded as she found other sources of social support.

In the family mentioned earlier where the grandmother thwarted efforts to encourage pain coping behaviors, we attempted to set up a family conference to discuss the child's pain management program with the extended family. However, the grandmother was unwilling to come in. Therefore, the mother decided to use a neighbor, rather than the grandmother, for after-school child care.

PROBLEM: THE ADULT'S PROBLEMATIC BEHAVIOR IS NEGATIVELY REINFORCED

Prevent Escape or Avoidance and Reinforce Adaptive Behaviors

This may be one of the most difficult family systems issues to address, since escape and avoidance can be such powerful reinforcers. Family therapy is needed in situations in which the parent is fostering pain or dependency or other maladaptive behaviors in the child in order to avoid their own problems. These family problems cannot be resolved unless the parent finds another way to deal with the aversive situation. For example, the parent who effectively avoids a stressful work situation by having a sick child may need help finding alternative solutions to his/her job difficulties. Similarly, the parent who avoids marital conflicts or avoids unwanted sexual relations by ministering to the sick child will need help finding alternative ways to resolve these conflicts. The clinician should be alert to the broader family perspective and be prepared to address the underlying issues that can thwart pain management efforts.

In some cases, the parent's maladaptive behaviors are negatively reinforced by a reduction in anxiety. Consider the following common example. The mother is afraid that her son's pain complaints signal a life-threatening condition and takes the child to the doctor for medical tests. The tests are negative, the mother is relieved, her anxiety diminishes. Thus, the mother's over-reaction to the child's pain complaints is negatively reinforced by the reduction in her anxiety that follows the medical testing. The solution to this problem is (1) for the medical staff to refuse to conduct further medical tests, and (2) for the psychologist to help the parent develop other ways to manage her anxiety about the child's condition. Cognitive strategies designed to confront the distortions in the parent's thinking would be helpful in this situation. A good collaboration with the medical team is essential if this intervention is to be successful. Unfortunately, it is often difficult to engage parents in psychotherapy and difficult to prevent them from "doctor shopping" until they find someone who will conduct the tests they request.

PROBLEM: APPROPRIATE ADULT BEHAVIOR IS INADEQUATELY REINFORCED OR PUNISHED

Prevent Punishment and Reinforce Appropriate Behavior

The mother of one young pain patient had attempted to help him distract himself when he was in pain. However, her husband repeatedly ridiculed her attempts and told her she was "incompetent." As a result, she had stopped trying to assist her son and felt increasingly embarrassed about her incompetence. Therapy for this family involved providing the mother with specific training in distraction skills and instructing the father to stop all critical comments to the mother and to praise at least one aspect of her handling of the child's pain each day. He also needed training in delivering praise before he could do so without sounding critical or sarcastic.

PROBLEM: THE ADULT LACKS THE SKILLS NEEDED TO DEAL MORE EFFECTIVELY WITH THE CHILD

Provide Skill Training

As the preceding example illustrates, parents often lack the skills necessary to help their child cope with pain or behave in a more adaptive fashion. One cannot assume that parents have good behavior management skills and will be able to praise or ignore their child's behavior appropriately. They may have no idea how to effectively use distraction for painful episodes. Or, they too may lack the listening skills necessary to communicate effectively with their child. Therefore, the clinician should be prepared to offer didactic instruction as well as model and role-play parenting skills as part of a comprehensive pain management intervention.

Implementing the Pain Management Program

Once a comprehensive conceptualization and treatment plan has been developed, the clinician should meet with the family and present the proposed treatment plan. This allows the clinician to be sure that the child, family, and health care team are in agreement with the goals of treatment and that all parties understand the expected course of treatment.

It is crucial that the treatment plan be framed in a way that the family can accept. At this point, the clinician should have a good enough understanding of the child and family to be able to discuss treatment options in a way that is compatible with the values and concerns of the child and family.

A typical format for a feedback and treatment planning session is presented in Table 14.1. After each topic in the table is discussed, the therapist should solicit comments, reactions, and impressions from the family. Any misunderstandings or disagreements in priorities or objectives should be addressed at this time. The actual intervention should not be initiated until the therapist and family have established a therapeutic contract and have agreed to the treatment plan. Important issues to address in this discussion are highlighted below.

In order to work together on a treatment plan, it is also essential that the family, clinician, and health care provider come to some agreement regarding the short- and long-term goals of treatment. For example, the child or family may expect total remission of pain, whereas the health care provider may believe that reducing the child's pain from severe to "mild" is the most appropriate goal of treatment. There

Table 14.1. Typical Format of a Feedback and Treatment Planning Session

I. Review of the reasons for referral
II. Explanation of the hypothesis generation testing process
III. Review of each primary hypothesis and findings obtained
IV. Summary of hypotheses supported by the data: Summary conceptualization
V. Presentation of treatment recommendations
VI. Determination of short-term and long-term treatment goals
VII. Determination of measurement strategies
VIII. Discussion of details of treatment
    A. Frequency of sessions
    B. Setting of sessions
    C. Participants
    D. Fees
    E. Confidentiality
IX. Initiation of treatment after all parties agree with treatment plan

is no point in proceeding with a psychological pain management program if some agreement regarding goals cannot be reached.

Similarly, the rate at which progress is expected should be presented. If it is likely to be several weeks or months before the child can return to school, this should be discussed. Family expectations that may be unrealistic or developmentally inappropriate should be addressed at this time.

Whenever possible, goals should reflect the family's and child's priorities. If being able to play baseball is a high priority for the child, one may get better compliance with rehabilitation if ball play is the goal and the reward, than if one just focuses on school attendance (which may be the therapist's or parents' top priority).

DETERMINE THE MEANS BY WHICH TREATMENT EFFICACY WILL BE MEASURED

The data collected in the course of the assessment process should suggest the most useful outcome measurement strategies. At the very minimum, the outcome assessment should incorporate the following basic measurement principles. The clinician should:

1 | Use multiple measures from multiple informants, to minimize bias.
2 | Use observational data whenever feasible.
3 | Measure behavior in multiple settings to ensure generalizability of findings.
4 | Tailor the measures to the quality and quantity of the individual child's pain. Do not try to apply a generic system to all children.

5 | Take repeated measures, so that fluctuations in symptoms can be measured.

6 | Make the measurement process as efficient as possible to maximize compliance. For example, a pain self-report form that is attached to the child's class schedule is more likely to be completed than a diary that is easily left at home.

7 | Reinforce compliance with outcome measurement. Be sure to discuss pain records at the beginning of each treatment session to communicate their importance (Meichenbaum & Turk, 1987).

PLAN AND IMPLEMENT THE PAIN MANAGEMENT INTERVENTION

The process of getting to this point may seem so complicated and cumbersome that one would never get the chance to actually implement a treatment program. However, when a clinician lets the pressures of the medical staff or the urgency of the family convince him/her to conduct a less than thorough evaluation or to truncate the baseline data collection, it almost always backfires. For example, without baseline data, the clinician is helpless when the treatment program is not progressing as well as was hoped. Without baseline data, it is very difficult to help parents see the bigger picture of the child's progress—that a momentary setback does not mean a total treatment failure. A hurried assessment often results in incomplete or less than optimal treatment plans that ultimately have to be altered. In the worst cases, superficial assessments merely serve to confirm the clinician's biases and preferences and often result in the same "blanket" treatment being applied to all patients. In contrast, thorough case conceptualizations based on adequate baseline data may require revisions along the way, but are much less likely to be total treatment failures.

The Treatment Planning Worksheet in Appendix B offers a structure for planning the different components of treatment that will be needed to address each supported hypothesis. The Treatment Planning Worksheet also includes a section for noting briefly the results of the treatment evaluation.

Include Plans for Maintenance and Generalization of Treatment Effects

Any pain management treatment plan should include specific plans to ensure that the beneficial results of treatment will generalize to all relevant aspects of the child's life and that the benefits will be as long-lasting as possible. To accomplish these ends, treatment plans should include training the child to deal with multiple settings and situations, turning over therapist roles to others in the child's natural environment as soon as is feasible, and moving from contrived reinforcers to naturally occurring reinforcers (Stokes & Baer, 1977).

CONDUCT AN ONGOING EVALUATION OF
TREATMENT EFFECTIVENESS

The measurement of treatment effectiveness will most likely rely on ongoing measurement of pain behaviors (subjective and/or objective) as well as the desired adaptive behaviors the clinician wants to increase. These outcome indices should be tailored to the individual child, to be sure that they are valid and sensitive. For example, number of days of school attended may ultimately be an excellent index of long-term treatment effectiveness, but would not be likely to be a sensitive measure for a child with such severe pain that he/she is bedridden. A more appropriate immediate outcome measure might be number of hours per day out of bed. In the headache literature, children typically are asked to keep a headache diary in which they record headache frequency, duration, intensity, medication intake, and school attendance. Hermann, Blanchard, and Flor (1997) used the diary data to evaluate treatment effectiveness by calculating the percent reduction in a Headache Index (which was calculated by "summing headache hours multiplied by the respective headache intensity across all headache episodes" [p. 612]).

For monitoring acute pain during medical procedures, the Observation Scale of Behavioral Distress (OSBD) (Jay, Ozolins, Elliott, & Caldwell, 1983) is the most widely used instrument in the research literature. The OSBD consists of verbal, vocal, and motor indicators of pain and distress. Typically, the child is videotaped during the medical procedure. A trained observer then codes the presence or absence of each OSBD behavior during each 15-second interval on the tape. A summary distress score is then created for the procedure by summing across all intervals, multiplying the behavior score by a predetermined intensity weight, and then dividing by the number of observation intervals. The resulting weighted mean distress score per interval can be used to monitor the child's progress over the course of treatment.

The OSBD has many advantages. Since it is widely used, findings can easily be compared to the literature and to scores obtained at other pain management programs. The scores also seem to be sensitive to clinical pain management interventions (e.g., Dahlquist et al., 1985, 1986; Jay & Eilliott, 1990; Jay, Elliott, Katz, & Siegel, 1987). However, the interval coding used in the OSBD is very time-intensive and highly trained observers are needed. Thus, the OSBD may not be a practical measure to use in non-research settings.

Long-Term Impact

To assess the more long-term impact of treatment on the child's day-to-day functioning, the clinician should consider the impact of improved pain management on the following important areas of children's functioning:

1	Academic performance
2	Social interactions with peers
3	Adaptive functioning/degree of disability, and
4	General emotional status, behavior problems, family harmony, etc.

Academic Functioning

Academic performance can be measured simply in terms of the number of complete days of school attended. It may be even more informative to also assess academic achievement (i.e., grades, test scores, progress through the curriculum, etc.). More effective pain management should enable the child to attend school more often and therefore make better academic progress.

Social Interactions with Peers

In general, physical illnesses can limit the amount and/or types of interactions children have with their peers (LaGreca, 1990). Physically ill children may not interact with peers as often as their healthy counterparts for a number of reasons (e.g., pain, physical impairment, parental concerns, or social withdrawal) (Miller, 1993). They also may have a smaller peer network (i.e., a smaller number of different peers with whom they interact) (Pendley, Dahlquist, & Dreyer, 1997; Pendley, Dahlquist, Cradock, & Warren, 1996). If social interactions are too restricted, children will not have the opportunity to develop friendships and learn important peer interaction skills (Harper, 1991). Improvement in the child's pain should enable the child to engage in a greater amount of interaction with peers.

We developed the Peer Interaction Record (PIR) (Thompson, Power, & Dahlquist, 1998) to provide a simple method for assessing the frequency of children's social interactions with peers. This measure, which is presented in Appendix C, is a 15-minute structured interview in which the child or parent is asked how many times the child has engaged in various activities with peers over the previous week. The items constituting the PIR were adapted from the Health and Daily Living Form (Moos, Cronkite, Billings, & Finney, 1984) and from Zarbatany, Hartmann, and Rankin's (1990) survey of the most common activites of 5th and 6th grade children. The PIR also allows the clinician to calculate the number of different peers with whom the child interacts (i.e., the size of the child's peer network).

There are many other aspects of social adjustment, social competence, and social skill that may be positively affected by increased interactions with peers, and thus could be thought of as second-order long-term benefits of improved pain. See Recommended Readings for summaries of this extensive literature.

Adaptive Functioning/Degree of Disability

If the child's pain condition improves, one also would expect the child to be able to resume a greater proportion of normal physical and self-help activities. Thus, one would expect to see improvements in physical capacities, such as strength and stamina, which could be ascertained from repeated assessments made by a physical therapist. Improvements in functional status or functional capacity (e.g., the child's ability to perform age-appropriate activities) (Stein, Gortmaker, Perrin, Pless, Walker, & Weitzman, 1987) also should follow improved pain status. There are a variety of measures that have been used in the literature. Some are general rating systems which classify the child's overall functional status. For example, the Chronic Activity Limitations Scale (CALS) classifies children into four categories based on their functional capacity (Lovell, 1992).

Class 1	Unable to engage in school or play activity appropriate for their age group;
Class 2	Limited in amount or type of primary activity (requires adapted school or play);
Class 3	Limited in minor activities (e.g., athletics); and
Class 4	Not limited in any activity.

However, global systems such as this one are unlikely to be sensitive to important changes in functional status that may occur within these large categories (Lovell, 1992; Murray & Passo, 1995).

Another global rating system, The Play Performance Scale for Children (Lansky, et al., 1987) makes a few more discriminations in the level of activity demonstrated by the child. To complete the scale, a rater indicates from the list below the single category that best reflects the child's average performance over the past week.

100	Fully active, normal
90	Minor restrictions in physically strenuous activity
80	Active, but tires more quickly
70	Both greater restriction of, and less time spent in, active play
60	Up and around but minimal active play; keeps busy with quieter activities
50	Gets dressed, but lies around much of the day; no active play; able to participate in all quiet play and activities
40	Mostly in bed; participates in quiet activities
30	In bed; needs assistance even for quiet play
20	Often sleeping; play entirely limited to very passive activities
10	No play; does not get out of bed
0	Unresponsive (Lansky et al., 1987, p. 1656)

Based on the content of these items, the Play Performance Scale for children may be most applicable to children with severe postoperative pain or severe disease pain. It also should be noted that, since the magnitude of the differences between each of these levels has not been validated, this scale is should be used as an ordinal rather than an interval scale.

The Juvenile Arthritis Functional Assessment Scale (JAFAS) (Lovell et al., 1989) is a more sensitive measure of the child's ability to perform ten motor and self-help tasks while a professional observes and times the performance. Although the reliability and validity of the measure is good, the JAFAS may be impractical to use in some settings, because it requires standardized equipment and trained personnel to administer (Murray & Passo, 1995).

The self-report format of the Juvenile Arthritis Functional Assessment Report (JAFAR) (Howe et al., 1991) can be used without specialized training. Parents and children complete separate forms of this scale, indicating how often (all the time, sometimes, or almost never) the child was able to perform 23 physical tasks over the past week.

The Childhood Health Assessment Questionnaire (Singh, Arthreya, Fries, & Goldsmith, 1994) also includes a disability section in which parents or children 8 years of age and older rate the child's functioning in eight areas (see Table 14.2). Two estimates are obtained: (1) how much difficulty the child experiences performing each task, and (2) how much assistance the child requires in completing the task.

Finally, it may be useful to measure concomitant improvements in more general aspects of the child's and the child's family's functioning following pain interventions. For example, it may be reasonable to see decreases in the child's depression or anxiety, decreased parenting stress, and fewer behavior problems at home or at school. For comprehensive reviews of assessment strategies for these broader aspects of children's functioning see Mash and Terdal (1997).

Re-Evaluation

If the treatment program is not working as expected, the conceptualization of the child's pain problem as well as the treatment plan must be re-evaluated. New hypotheses should be generated to explain why the program is not working. For example, the initial goals may have been too high, the intervention strategies may not be appropriate for this child, the selected reinforcers may be inadequate, the parents may not be following recommendations, or skill deficits may have been overlooked. The original hypotheses should be re-examined and new hypotheses added as appropriate.

For example, when the child's pain problem appears relatively straightforward, but straightforward pain management strategies are not working, it is often the case that larger family/systemic factors that were overlooked in the initial conceptualization are interfering with the intervention. If so, the factors maintaining

Table 14.2. Functional Capacities Assessed by the Childhood Health Assessment Questionnaire

Standing/walking

- Stand up from a low chair
- Get in and out of bed
- Walk outdoors on flat ground
- Climb up five steps

Reach

- Reach up and get down a heavy object
- Bend down to pick up something off the floor
- Pull sweater on over head
- Turn neck to look back over shoulder

Eating

- Cut meat
- Lift a cup or glass to mouth
- Open a new cereal box

Grip

- Write or scribble with pen or pencil
- Open car doors
- Turn faucets on or off
- Turn a door knob and push open a door

Dressing and grooming

- Dress, tie shoelaces, do buttons
- Shampoo hair
- Remove socks
- Cut fingernails

Hygiene

- Wash and dry entire body
- Take a tub bath (get in and out of tub)
- Get on and off the toilet
- Brush teeth
- Comb/brush hair

Activities

- Run errands and shop
- Get in and out of car or school bus
- Ride bike
- Do household chores (wash dishes, take out trash, vacuum, make bed)
- Run and play

the parents' or child's behaviors should be examined more closely. One 12-year-old child with stomach pain refused to return to school. There was no apparent physical etiology for the pain complaints. Although a reward program had been in place for a few weeks, she continued to remain at home in bed, claiming she was too ill to attend school. In one therapy session, the frustrated psychologist was trying to help her see the importance of going on with her life despite her pain. By way of example, the psychologist said, "Your mother can't just go to bed and stop taking care of the house or the family if she gets a headache ..." The girl interrupted, saying, "Oh yes she can! She does it all the time! She didn't cook at all yesterday!" It turned out that the mother had not been enforcing the behavioral program because to do so would also invalidate *her own* maladaptive pain behavior. As a result of this new information, the therapy focus shifted and a more comprehensive evaluation of the family system was conducted.

REVISE THE TREATMENT PLAN IF NECESSARY

Based on a re-examination of the data and the generation and testing of new hypotheses, the treatment plan should be revised if necessary. New data should be

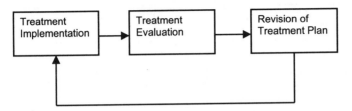

Figure 14.1. The cycle of treatment implementation, evaluation, and revision.

collected and treatment effectiveness re-evaluated. As illustrated in Figure 14.1, this cycle of implementation, evaluation, and revision repeats until the problem is successfully treated.

—————————————————————————————— CASE EXAMPLE

To illustrate how the various components of this conceptualization framework fit together in the formulation of a single case, we will conclude with a brief summary of a patient who was evaluated and subsequently treated for arthromyalgia and stomach aches of unknown etiology. Figure 14.2 shows the hypotheses that were generated, the evaluation plan, and the main findings (i.e., which hypotheses were supported).

——————————————————————————— Presenting Problem

Kim, a 9-year-old girl, was referred by a pediatric gastroenterologist for pain management. According to medical records, Kim began complaining of pain in her stomach, limbs, and joints about 7 months prior to referral, at around the start of the school year. She missed more than 10 full days of school during the preceding 6 months due to these problems. In addition, she frequently felt sick at school and went home early.

She was evaluated by a gastroenterologist and appeared to have lactose intolerance; however her symptoms persisted despite a lactose-free diet. A rheumatologist also had evaluated her, but found no organic cause for her symptoms. Kim and her mother said that the physicians told them that stress might be causing some of Kim's symptoms.

Although Kim occasionally had problems with allergies in the past, she had no problems the past school year. She was not taking any prescription or nonprescription medications. She had no history of other medical illnesses. According to the referring physician, her medical evaluation was unremarkable.

The information summarized above was obtained from the physician when she phoned in the referral and from a brief conversation with Kim's mother to ex-

Physical hypotheses	Sources of data	Evaluation plan	Test results
1. Is the child receiving less than optimal pain medication?	Parent interview Child interview Medical staff interview	Mother interview Father interview Child interview Medical staff interview	1. *Possibly* No prescription or over-the-counter pain medication used
2. Are medications administered inappropriately?	Chart review Medication records Observe child		2. *NA*
3. Is the child failing to get all scheduled medication doses?	Pain diaries: child and parent		3. *NA*
4. Are pain medications unavailable?			4. *NA*
5. Are other physical factors exacerbating the child's pain? • *Protective posturing?* • *Muscle tension?* • *Fatigue?* • *Environmental factors?* • *Over-exertion?* • *PT Noncompliance?*	Parent interview Medical staff interview Observation of child Pain Diaries: child and parent	Mother interview Father interview Medical staff interview Observation of child	5. *Some support,* see below • *Not supported.* No protective posturing evident. • *Probable muscle tension.* No data, but reports high anxiety. • *Probable fatigue.* Bedtime is late for age. • *No data* • *Not supported.* Not related to activity. • *NA*

Cognitive/emotional hypotheses	Sources of data	Evaluation plan	Test results
1. Is the child's attention focused on the pain?	Child interview Parent interview Medical staff interview (MD, RN, therapist) Teacher interview	1. Child interview 2. Parent interview Child pain diary Parent pain records Teacher interview	1. *Supported.* Spends much time talking with mother about pain or worrying about having pain.
2. Is anxiety or stress exacerbating the child's pain? • Are aspects of the child's environment frightening? • Are clear signals for the onset and termination of painful stimuli lacking? • Does the pain increase under stressful conditions?	Observation Child pain diary Parent pain records	1. Child interview 2. Parent interview Child pain diary Parent pain records Teacher interview	2. *Supported.* • *Not supported.* Doesn't appear frightened at school or home. (Check further: Possible frightening marital conflict?) • *NA* • *Supported.* Pain occurs primarily in the morning, on school days, during school, or at night when talking about worries and school concerns. Also greater at times of conflict with mother and sister.

Figure 14.2. Case conceptualization example, hypothesis generation, and evaluation planning worksheet.

Cognitive/emotional hypotheses	Sources of data	Evaluation plan	Test results
3. Does the child engage in self-defeating thinking about the pain?	Child Interview Parent interview	1. Child interview 2. Observation 3. Parent interview	3. *Supported.* Extremely negative self-statements in a variety of situations. Says she can't do academic tasks, gives up without effort, negative comments about tasks, negative comments about self, appearance, lack of friends, poor chances of future academic or social success.
4. Does the pain have significant meaning for the child?	Child interview	1. Child interview Child pain diary	4. *Supported.* Pain complaints seem to represent underlying emotional distress (sadness, anger, frustration, anxiety). Seems to signal need to talk to someone, get reassurance, support.
5. Is the caregiver's emotional or cognitive status interfering?	Parent interview Observation Medical staff interview Child interview	1. Parent interview	5. *Not known but possible.* Mother reports being nervous herself, insomnia problems, also hints at marital conflict. Plan: continue to assess.

Behavioral hypotheses	Sources of data	Evaluation plan	Test results
1. Is the child's pain behavior positively reinforced?	Home observation School observation Clinic observation Child's pain diary Parent pain records Teacher pain records Parental interview Child interview Teacher interview School nurse interview Counselor interview	1. Parental interview 2. Child interview Parent pain records Child pain diary Teacher interview School nurse interview School observation	1. *Supported.* Gets attention and reassurance from mother, time alone talking with mother, mother stays home from work, mother sleeps with her, rubs her back.

2. Is the child's pain behavior negatively reinforced?	Same as 1.	1. Parental interview 2. Child Interview Parental pain records Child pain diary Teacher interview School nurse interview School observation	2. *Supported.* Avoids going to school. Able to leave school. Avoids conflicts with mother. Diminished anxiety after talking with mother.
3. Is adaptive behavior inadequately reinforced or punished?	Same as 1.	1. Parental interview 2. Child interview Parental pain records Teacher interview School nurse interview School observation	3. *Supported.* Younger sister is a "star," gets lots of kudos socially and academically. Kim doesn't get much attention for positives. School is difficult, perhaps too difficult. Mom spends long hours at work when Kim is well.
4. Does the child lack the skills necessary to perform the adaptive behavior? • Cognitive/academic deficits?	Intelligence tests Achievement tests Academic tests Neuropsychological tests	1. WISC-R 2. Review of recent achievement test given at school	4. *Partially supported.* • *Partially supported.* IQ fine: VIQ = 128, PIQ=128, FSIQ = 131 (97th percentile) Achievement testing: 80th percentiles in math; 90th percentiles in all other areas. No apparent deficits. Anxiety interfered with performance, esp. auditory memory. Easily frustrated—gave up on difficult items. Careless.

Figure 14.2. (*Continued*)

Behavioral hypotheses	Sources of data	Evaluation plan	Test results
• Social/Communication deficits?	Child interview Parental interview Teacher interview Counselor interview Observe at school and home	1. Child interview 2. Parent interview	• Supported. Only talks with mother about concerns after pain complaints. Frequent fights with her mother. Feels unattractive, thinks others don't like her.
5. Is the adult's problematic behavior positively reinforced?	Home observation Clinic observation Child's pain diary Parent pain records Parent interview Child interview Medical staff interview	1. Parent pain records 2. Parent interview Home/clinic observation Medical staff interview	5. Not supported. No evidence at this time.
6. Is the adult's problematic behavior negatively reinforced?	Same as 5.	1. Parent pain records 2. Parent interview Home/clinic observation Medical staff interview	6. Supported. Mother does not like her job, would like to quit, conflicts with boss. Kim stops temper tantrums when allowed to stay home, calms down when allowed to come home from school.
7. Is appropriate adult behavior inadequately reinforced or punished?	Same as 5.	1. Parent pain records 2. Parent interview Home/clinic observation Medical staff interview	7. Supported. Kim throws temper tantrums, sobs when mother tries to make her go to school.

Figure 14.2. (*Continued*)

plain the evaluation process and set up the initial interview. Based on this information, we generated the hypotheses presented in Figure 14.2 and established a preliminary evaluation plan. Numbered items in the Evaluation Plan column indicate the initial assessments that were planned. Unnumbered items indicate alternate strategies to be used if the initial methods did not yield adequate data.

Since parent interviews appeared to have the potential to provide data regarding several of the hypotheses, the parent interview was conducted first, followed by an interview with the child later the same day. The interviews provided extensive information related to many of the hypotheses.

Kim is the eldest of two children. She has a younger sister, age 6. Her mother works as a receptionist. Her father is a high school science teacher. The parents have been married for 10 years.

Kim attends the local elementary school, where she is enrolled in the gifted and talented program. This is the first year she has been enrolled in the program, which is a self-contained accelerated third grade classroom. According to her parents and school records, her development has always been advanced for her age. She reportedly began talking at 6.5 months, walked at 9 months, and potty-trained herself at 18 months. Her school achievement tests consistently placed her well above her grade level. For example, she scored at the sixth grade level in math concepts in first grade and at the fifth grade level in vocabulary.

Both parents described Kim as a "worrier." She is extremely afraid of water and the dark. She says she is unattractive and too skinny and complains that she is not as pretty as her best friend or her sister. Some nights she lies awake reportedly worrying about world peace. She and her mother frequently argue about her failure to go to sleep at an appropriate time. Many school nights she is awake until midnight.

With respect to schoolwork, she is a "perfectionist," according to her parents. She is not satisfied with her work unless she obtains the best grade in her class. She insists on striving for straight A's, even though her parents have told her that lower grades would be fine. She insists that she must have all A's in order to get a college scholarship.

Kim did not have any pain problems prior to the present school year. She missed four days of school in October because of the flu, but has not had any other illnesses. Currently, she complains of pain every night at bedtime. Her mother lies down with her and talks with her when she is not feeling well. She rubs her back and tries to help her relax, but reports that this does not appear to help. Changing her diet to exclude milk products also does not seem to have helped.

Kim also complains of pain on most school days. Over the past month she has missed at least one day per week because she was in too much pain to go to school. She also has come home from school early every day this month because of pain. She typically calls her mother between 10:00 and 11:00 A.M. and is picked up as soon as her mother can get there. At home, she and her mother work on her homework or Kim lies on the couch watching TV. However, on the weekends, she seems to have more energy and plays with friends in the neighborhood.

Her mother reported that she does not like her boss, so it is a bit of a relief to get out of the office to care for Kim. However, she is getting in trouble for missing so much work. She is afraid that she may lose her job if her attendance does not improve. The family needs the extra income and cannot afford for her to quit. Both parents reported that they personally have problems sleeping. Her mother acknowledged that she tends to be "nervous" also.

In the initial interview, Kim appeared guarded. She offered only brief answers and seemed to look for a reaction from the clinician, as if to see if she had given the "correct" answer. She did not laugh or smile and made poor eye contact. Nonetheless, several important pieces of information were obtained.

Kim described her pain in very vague terms. She described an achy feeling like someone is "pulling" on her thighs and upper arms. She also said her stomach hurts. She said the pain varies weekly and tends to be the worst in the mornings and afternoons. Tylenol® and aspirin do not relieve the pain. Soaking in a warm bath has helped very slightly. Heating pads provide no help. Rubbing on the affected area feels "good," but the pain does not go away.

Kim acknowledged that she "had always had stomach problems," and that anything that makes her startled or worried can make the pain worse. For example, she said she always has a stomach ache on the first day of school, and when she goes to the doctor or dentist. She reported that scary movies and her parents' fighting cause her stomach to hurt. School also makes her stomach hurt, although she wasn't exactly sure what about school worries her.

According to Kim, she and her mother fight a lot. They argue about her grades, her temper, fights with her sister, and chores. She said her mother does not hit her, but yells a lot. Her father, according to Kim, tends to be quieter, but quick to spank. Kim was unable to describe any efforts on her part to lessen the conflicts with her mother. She seemed to have no idea about any other ways to handle conflict other than yelling, cussing, kicking, throwing things, and hitting.

Because many of Kim's pain symptoms appeared related to school, formal cognitive testing was conducted and school achievement records were reviewed to rule out cognitive or academic deficits. Kim obtained a Verbal Scale IQ score of 128, a Performance Scale IQ score of 128, and a Full Scale IQ score of 131 on the Wechsler Intelligence Scale for Children–Revised (WISC-R). Her scores fell within the 97–98th percentiles and are considered in the superior to very superior range of intellectual functioning.

Kim performed well above average on most of the WISC-R subtests, with striking strengths in her general fund of knowledge. However, she performed relatively poorly on tests of short-term auditory recall of digits. She appeared extremely anxious on this subtest, fidgeting and making frequent negative comments about her performance. She also responded quickly with no apparent efforts to check her work on several visual–motor tasks. This carelessness resulted in lowered scores on several subtests.

A review of her academic records revealed above average performance in math and superior level performance in all other subjects. Her most recent report card listed her grades as all A's.

On the State-Trait Anxiety Inventory for Children (STAIC) (Spielberger, Edwards, Lushene, Monturi, & Platzek, 1973), Kim denied any feelings of state anxiety (T score = 35), but reported elevated trait anxiety (T score = 70). On the Children's Depression Inventory (CDI) (Kovacs & Beck, 1977), she obtained a score of 13. Most of the items she endorsed involved feeling bothered and worrying, experiencing aches and pains, getting into trouble, and feeling unattractive, rather than more depressive symptoms.

Conceptualization

The results of the evaluation were entered on the Hypothesis Generation and Evaluation Planning worksheet, presented in Figure 14.3. In brief, the evaluation supported the following conceptualization.

Physical Factors

Since Kim was not taking any medications, it is possible that she was not receiving optimal pain medication. However, given the variable and sporadic nature of her symptoms and the vagueness of her report, medication did not appear to be the optimal intervention at this time. Furthermore, the nonsteroidal medications she had tried so far had not helped (aspirin and Tylenol®). Therefore, further action on medication hypotheses was deferred. However, the evaluation did suggest that muscle tension and fatigue were likely to be exacerbating her pain problem. She was not getting adequate sleep for her age and she reported a high level of anxiety that is likely to be associated with muscle tension.

Cognitive Emotional Factors

Almost all of the cognitive hypotheses were supported. Kim's pain appeared to be related to stressful situations. She had pain primarily before or during school, when talking about worries and when involved in or witnessing family conflict. She focused considerable attention on her symptoms. Her pain symptoms also seem to serve an important function of engaging her mother in extended discussions of her emotional concerns. Thus, the pain may have been be her way of communicating her emotional needs to her mother.

Physical hypotheses	Test results	Treatment plan
1. Is the child receiving less than optimal pain medication?	Possibly	Wait for now. Medication may not be necessary.
2. Are medications administered inappropriately?	NA	
3. Is the child failing to get all scheduled medication doses?	NA	
4. Are pain medications unavailable?	NA	
5. Are other physical factors exacerbating the child's pain?	Probable muscle tension / Probable fatigue	Teach progressive muscle relaxation to combat muscle tension when stressed or anxious and facilitate falling asleep. Set earlier bedtime. Enforce independent falling asleep. / Discuss worries and concerns at a time other than bedtime.
Cognitive/emotional hypotheses	Test results	Treatment plan
1. Is the child's attention focused on the pain?	Supported	Restrict time spent talking about pain to a structured "Worry Time" each day.
2. Is anxiety or stress exacerbating the child's pain?	Supported	Minimize stress at school—alter expectations for perfection, clarify strengths and weaknesses with teachers, improve social skills. / Teach anxiety management skills (cognitive plus relaxation). / Reduce conflict with mother and sister and increase positive interactions with mother and sister. / Teach anger management skills. / Restrict time spent talking about worries to a structured "Worry Time" each day.

	Test results	Treatment plan
3. *Does the child engage in self-defeating thinking about the pain?*	Supported	Initiate cognitive therapy to challenge and teach ways to combat negative self-statements. Teach problem-solving strategies to replace helpless, catastrophic cognitions and giving up. Set more realistic expectations regarding academic success and social success. Provide social skills training as needed (e.g., conflict resolution skills).
4. *Does the pain have significant meaning for the child?*	Supported	Provide more direct ways for Kim to communicate concerns to her parents (e.g., through structured "Worry Time"). Prohibit discussion of worries at pain times.
5. *Is the caregiver's emotional or cognitive status interfering?*	Not known. Possible	Continue to assess mother's emotional status, possible marital conflict.
Behavioral hypotheses	**Test results**	**Treatment plan**
1. *Is the child's pain behavior positively reinforced?*	Supported	Restrict time spent talking about pain to one period per day. Do not conduct intimate discussions of feelings or worries after any pain reports. Ignore pain verbalizations at times other than Worry Time. Restrict Kim to bedroom with the lights out, no TV, no special activities if she misses school. Kim should fall asleep alone. No back rubs, etc.
2. *Is the child's pain behavior negatively reinforced?*	Supported	Kim should go to school and stay in school despite pain. Coordinate with MD and school officials. Ignore pain complaints. Require chores and enforce consequences for misbehavior despite pain. Teach alternative strategies to reduce anxiety (relaxation and cognitive) and get reassurance (Worry Time conversations with mother).

Figure 14.3. Case conceptualization example: Treatment planning worksheet.

Behavioral hypotheses	Test results	Treatment plan
3. Is adaptive behavior inadequately reinforced or punished?	Supported	Establish positive reinforcement program that recognizes Kim's accomplishments. Set realistic goals for school performance based on level of skill. Consult with teacher. Praise grades that meet these standards. Reward daily school attendance with daily special time with mother. Reward cooperative interactions with sister; compliance with mother's requests. Trade points for family outings on weekend.
4. Does the child lack the skills necessary to perform the adaptive behavior?	Partially supported	Provide training in the following skills: anxiety management (academic and social) (relaxation and cognitive strategies). Problem-solving for difficult academic problems, accuracy checking, self-monitoring. Communication skills (both Kim and mother), including listening, compromise. Social problem-solving skills for conflict situations with peers and parents. Peer initiation skills if needed.
5. Is the adult's problematic behavior positively reinforced?	Not supported	
6. Is the adult's problematic behavior negatively reinforced?	Supported	Have father deal with calls to come home from school. Ask school nurse to enforce a return to classroom rather than calling home. Explore alternative employment options with mother.
7. Is appropriate adult behavior inadequately reinforced or punished?	Supported	Support and praise mother's handling of pain behaviors in therapy sessions. Have father also praise efforts. Enlist father's aid in sending child to school despite pain complaints.

Figure 14.3. (*Continued*)

She also had many self-defeating thoughts about herself, her abilities, her health, and her appearance. He negative attitudes also were reflected in giving up on challenging cognitive tasks. She also set unrealistically high standards for herself.

Although less is known about her mother, there is some suggestion that she, too, was anxious. There also appeared to be some marital conflict. The degree to which these emotional issues interfered with the parent's ability to help her daughter cannot yet be determined.

Behavioral Factors

Kim appeared to receive considerable positive attention from her mother for her pain complaints. Her mother spent more time with her, slept with her, rubbed her back, and talked extensively with her about her worries. Negative reinforcement contingencies also were apparent in her ability to avoid attending school and escape from school via pain complaints. More indirectly, pain complaints resulted in extended conversations with her mother about her worries. After such conversations, it is reasonable to assume that she might have experienced a reduction in anxiety, which would negatively reinforce pain behavior. It is also possible that pain complaints might have helped avoid conflicts with her mother. Finally, it appeared that her adaptive efforts (i.e., school attendance, pain-free times, and other appropriate behaviors) received little positive attention.

Although her overall cognitive skills and academic achievement appeared excellent, Kim did appear to lack certain skills that would make her successful in school. Her high anxiety interfered with performance. She was easily frustrated and careless. She appeared to have poor problem-solving skills with which to approach challenging tasks.

In the social arena, her anxiety again was evident. Moreover, she and her mother appeared to have poor conflict resolution skills. She did not seem to know how to approach her mother to get support and nurturance without complaining of pain. She also had an overly negative view of her own attractiveness, which may have distorted her perceptions of other children's reactions to her. She also appeared to be lacking in basic peer initiation skills.

Her mother also may have lacked communication and conflict resolution skills, although this was not assessed directly. The most obvious contingencies that appeared to be maintaining her mother's behavior involved negative reinforcement. She appeared to be able to avoid her boss and her unpleasant job by inappropriately allowing Kim to stay home or to come home from school. The termination of Kim's complaints and tantrums when her mother gave in was another negative reinforcer. Her mother received little support or encouragement for sending Kim to school and considerable punishment in the form of aggression from Kim when she did try to make her go to school.

Treatment Plan

The treatment plan developed to address the hypotheses supported by the evaluation is presented in Figure 14.3. The desired behaviors for this youngster were conceptualized as: (1) communicating emotional concerns without using pain complaints, and (2) attending school daily for the entire day. Since the treatment recommendations are presented in considerable detail in the figure, they will not be reviewed again here. In general, the plan focused on cognitive restructuring, stress management and social skills training, and developing a contingency management program at home that would reinforce school attendance and the direct expression of emotional concerns and extinguish pain behaviors.

It should be noted that within this treatment plan the same intervention often served multiple purposes. For example, restricting the amount of time Kim discusses her worries to a single "Worry Time" appears in several places in the Treatment Plannning Worksheet. This particular intervention serves multiple functions. It keeps Kim's attention directed away from factors that exacerbate her pain, encourages a more direct expression of her worries without needing a pain symptom, encourages her mother to provide attention to Kim for something other than pain, provides opportunities for Kim and her mother to practice communication skills, minimizes inadvertent positive reinforcement of pain behaviors with intensive maternal attention, prevents the punishment of adaptive behavior by making sure Kim still had access to intimate conversations with her mother, and should help improve sleep, since she will not be talking about troubling issues right before she is supposed to go to sleep.

Treatment Outcome

From a pain management standpoint, the outcome of this case was remarkable. Pain complaints and hours of school attended were set as the outcome indices. Within three weeks, Kim was attending school the entire day every day. Pain complaints dropped to zero. Her mother and she were using the "Worry Time" technique after school every day and she was getting to sleep by 10:00 P.M. every night. However, Kim and her mother still were experiencing many daily conflicts. The focus of therapy, therefore, shifted to intensive communication and problem-solving training for Kim and her mother. A token reinforcement system was expanded to include daily chores and cooperative play with her sister. Kim continued to have many worries and to demonstrate negative thinking. These cognitive issues remained an ongoing focus of therapy as well.

15

Concluding Comments

As the scientific study of pharmacological and behavioral management of children's pain continues, new techniques for managing pain may emerge to be added to the repertoire of pain management strategies discussed in this book and in other pediatric pain management texts. Similarly, as our empirical base develops, the data may suggest that certain pain management strategies are superior to others for certain kinds of pain or for certain children in certain circumstances. For example, in our current research program, we are examining developmental and individual differences in parent–child interactions in order to try to more precisely match pain management interventions to the specific needs of the child and family. We hope to identify the parent–children pairs that will do best if provided ongoing professional support during painful medical procedures, versus those for whom training the parents to take over the pain management coaching role is most appropriate. We are also in the process of designing pain management techniques specifically for children with special needs, such as very young children and developmentally disabled children.

The clinicians who care for children with pain problems must continue to follow the literature to keep abreast of these and other developments in the relatively new field of pediatric pain management. However, the model of assessment and intervention presented here should not become outdated, since the process of hypothesis testing is not tied to any one set of data or to any specific interventions. The process of hypothesis generation, hypothesis testing, treatment planning, and treatment evaluation should remain applicable to pediatric pain management for many years to come.

References

American Psychiatric Association. (1994). *Diagnostic and statistical manual of mental disorders, (DSM-IV)* (4th ed.). Washington, DC: APA.

Allen, K. D., & Matthews, J. R. (1998). Behavior management of recurrent pain in children. In T. S. Watson & F. M. Gresham (Eds.), *Handbook of child behavior therapy* (pp. 263–285). New York: Plenum.

Allen, K. D., & McKeen, L. (1991). Home-based multicomponent treatment of pediatric migraine. *Headache, 31,* 467–472.

Bernstein, D. A., & Borkovec, T. D. (1973). *Progressive relaxation training: A manual for helping professions.* Champaign, IL. Research Press.

Blount, R. L., Bachanas, P. J., Powers, S. W., Cotter, M. W., Franklin, A., Chapplin, W., Mayfield, J., Henderson, M., & Blount, S.D. (1992). Training children to cope and parents to coach them during routine immunizations: Effects on child, parent, and staff behaviors. *Behavior Therapy, 23,* 689–705.

Blount, R. L., Dahlquist, L. M., Baer, R. A., & Wouri, D. (1984). A brief, effective method for teaching children to swallow pills. *Behavior Therapy, 15,* 381–387.

Blount, R. L., Davis, N., Powers, S., & Roberts, M. C. (1991). The influence of environmental factors and coping style on children's coping and distress. *Clinical Psychology Review, 11,* 93–116.

Blount, R. L., Powers, S. W., Cotter, M. W., Swan, S., & Free, K. (1994). Making the system work: Training pediatric oncology patients to cope and their parents to coach them during BMA/LP procedures. *Behavior Modification, 18,* 6–31.

Bush, J., & Cockrell, C. (1987). Maternal factors predicting parenting behaviors in the pediatric clinic. *Journal of Pediatric Psychology, 12,* 505–518.

Bush, J. P., & Harkins, S. W. (1991). *Children in pain: Clinical and research issues from a developmental perspective.* New York: Springer Verlag.

Bush, J. P., Holmbeck, G. N., & Cockrelli, J. L. (1989). Patterns of p.r.n. analgesic drug administration in children following elective surgery. *Journal of Pediatric Psychology, 14,* 433–448.

Cautela, J. R., & Groden, J. (1978). *Relaxation: A comprehensive manual for adults, children, and children with special needs.* Champaign, IL: Research Press.

Christensen, N. K., Terry, R. D., Wyatt, S., Pichert, J. W., & Lorenz, R. A. (1983). Quantitative assessment of dietary adherence in patients with insulin-dependent diabetes mellitus. *Diabetes Care, 6,* 245–250.

Dahlquist, L. M. (1990). Obtaining child reports in health care settings. In A. LaGreca (Ed.), *Child assessment: Through the eyes of the child* (pp. 395–439). Boston: Allyn and Bacon.

Dahlquist, L. M. (1992). Coping with aversive medical procedures. In A. M. LaGreca, L. J. Siegel, J. L. Wallander, & C. E. Walker (Eds.), *Advances in pediatric psychology: Stress and coping in child health* (pp. 345–376). New York: Guilford.

Dahlquist, L. M. (1997). Decreasing children's distress during cancer treatment. *In Session: Psychotherapy in Practice, 3,* 43–54.

Dahlquist, L. M., & Taub, E. (1991). Family adaptation to childhood cancer. In J. Vincent (Ed.), *Advances in family intervention, assessment, and theory* (Vol. 5, pp. 123–150). Greenwich, CT: JAI Press.

Dahlquist, L. M., Gil, K. M., Armstrong, F. D., DeLawyer, D. D., Greene, P., & Wuori, D. (1986). Preparing children for medical examinations: The importance of previous medical experience. *Health Psychology, 5,* 249–259.

Dahlquist, L. M., Gil, K., Armstrong, D., Ginsberg, A., & Jones, B. (1985). Behavioral management of children's distress during chemotherapy. *Journal of Behavior Therapy and Experimental Psychiatry, 16,* 325–329.

Dahlquist, L. M., Power, T. G., & Carlson, L. (1995). Physician and parent behavior during invasive cancer procedures: Relationships to child behavioral distress. *Journal of Pediatric Psychology, 20,* 477–490.

Dahlquist, L. M., Power, T. G., Cox, C. N., & Fernbach, D. J. (1994). Parenting and child distress during cancer procedures: A multidimensional assessment. *Children's Health Care, 23,* 149–166.

Dahlquist, L. M., Pendley, J. S., Landthrip, D. S., Jones, C. L., Steuber, C. P., & Wirtz, P. (1998). Reducing children's distress during invasive cancer procedures: The relative effectiveness of parent- versus therapist-delivered coaching in cognitive behavioral skills. Unpublished manuscript, University of Maryland Baltimore County.

Derrickson, J. G., Neef, N. A., & Cataldo, M. F. (1993). Effects of signaling procedures on a hospitalized infant's affective behavior. *Journal of Applied Behavior Analysis, 26,* 133–134.

Drotar, D. (1995). Consulting with pediatricians: Psychological perspectives. New York: Plenum.

Elliott, C. H., & Olson, R. A. (1983). The management of children's distress in response to painful medical treatment for burn injuries. *Behaviour Research and Therapy, 21,* 675–683.

Ferber, R. (1985). *Solve your child's sleep problems.* New York: Simon & Schuster.

Fordyce, W. E. (1976). *Behavioral methods for chronic pain and illness.* St. Louis, MO: Mosby.

Forehand, R., & McMahon, R. (1981). *Helping the noncompliant child: A clinician's guide to parent training.* New York: Guilford.

Funk, M. J., Mullins, L. L., & Olson, R. A. (1984). Teaching children to swallow pills: A case study. *Children's Health Care, 13,* 20–23.

Gelfand, D., & Hartman, D. H. (1984). *Child behavior analysis and therapy* (2nd ed.). New York: Pergamon.

Gelfand, K., Dahlquist, L. M., & Hass, J. M. (1998). Parental nonverbal behavior and child distress during painful medical procedures. Unpublished manuscript, University of Maryland Baltimore County.

Gelfand, K., Pringle, B., Senuta, K., Hilley, L., Dahlquist, L. M., & Eskenazi, A. (November 1998). *Distress management for pediatric chemotherapy: Addressing environmental challenges.* Poster presented at the Association for the Advancement of Behvavior Therapy, Washington, DC.

Gil, K. M., Thompson, R. J., Keith, B. R., Tota-Faucette, M., Noll, S., & Kinney, T. R. (1993). Sickle cell disease pain in children and adolescents: Change in pain frequency and coping strategies over time. *Journal of Pediatric Psychology, 18,* 621–637.

Gil, K. M., Williams, D. A., Thompson, Jr., R. J., & Kinney, T. R. (1991). Sickle cell disease in children and adolescents: The relation of child and parent pain coping strategies to adjustment. *Journal of Pediatric Psychology, 16,* 643–663.

Gil, K. M., Wilson, J. J., Edens, J. L., Workman, E., Ready, J., Sedway, J., Reading-Lallinger, R., & Daeschner, C. W. (in press). Cognitive coping skills training in children with sickle cell disease pain. *International Journal of Behavioral Medicine.*

Harper, D. C. (1991). Paradigms for investigating rehabilitation and adaptation to childhood disability and chronic illness. *Journal of Pediatric Psychology, 16,* 533–542.

Hermann, C., Blanchard, E. B., & Flor, H. (1997). Biofeedback treatment for pediatric migraine: Prediction of treatment outcome. *Journal of Consulting and Clinical Psychology, 65,* 611–616.

Hilley, L. & Dahlquist, L. M. (1998). The role of parental support behaviors as mediators of child distress. Unpublished manuscript, University of Maryland Baltimore County.

Howe, S., Levinson, J., Shear, E., Hartner, S., McGirr, G., Schulte, M., & Lovell, D. (1991). Development of a disability measurement tool for juvenile rheumatoid arthritis: The Juvenile Arthritis Functional Assessment Report for Children and Their Parents. *Arthritis and Rheumatism, 34,* 873–880.

Hughes, J. N., & Baker, D. B. (1990). *The clinical child interview.* New York: Guilford.

Jay, S. M., & Elliott, C. H. (1990). A stress inoculation program for parents whose children are undergoing painful medical procedures. *Journal of Consulting and Clinical Psychology, 58,* 799–804.

Jay, S. M., Elliott, C. H., Katz, E., & Siegel, S. E. (1987). Cognitive–behavioral and pharmacologic interventions for children's distress during painful medical procedures. *Behaviour Research and Therapy, 23,* 513–520.

Jay, S. M., Elliott, C. H., Woody, P. D., & Siegel, S. E. (1991). An investigation of cognitive–behavioral therapy combined with oral Valium for children undergoing medical procedures. *Health Psychology, 10,* 317–322.

Jay, S. M., Ozolins, M., Elliott, C. H., & Caldwell, S. (1983). Assessment of children's distress during painful medical procedures. *Health Psychology, 2,* 133–147.

Johnson, J. E., Kirchoff, K. T., & Endress, M. P. (1975). Altering children's distress behavior during orthopedic cast removal. *Nursing Research, 24,* 404–410.

Johnson, S. B., Silverstein, J. H., Rosenbloom, A. L., Carter, R., & Cunningham, W. (1986). Assessing daily management in childhood diabetes. *Health Psychology, 5,* 545–564.

Kendall, P. C. (Ed.). (1991). Child and adolescent therapy: Cognitive–behavioral procedures. New York: Guilford.

Kopp, C. B. (1982). Antecedents of self-regulation: A developmental perspective. *Developmental Psychology, 18,* 199–214.

Kovacs, M., & Beck, A. (1977). An empirical clinical approach towards a definition of childhood depression. In J. G. Schulterbrandt & A. Raskin (Eds.), *Depression in children. Diagnosis, treatment and conceptual models* (pp. 1–25). New York: Raven Press.

Kunz, J. R. M., & Finkel, A. J. (Eds.). (1987). *The American Medical Association family medical guide.* New York: Random House.

LaGreca, A. M. (Ed.). (1990). *Through the eyes of the child: Obtaining child reports from children and adolescents.* New York: Allyn & Bacon.

Landthrip, D. S., Pendley, J. S., Dahlquist, L. M., & Jones, C. L. (November 1994). *Practical, cost-effective anxiety management intervention for preschool children undergoing cancer treatment.* Paper presented at the annual meeting of the Association for the Advancement of Behavior Therapy, San Diego, CA.

Lansky, S. B., List, M. A., Lansky, L. L., & Ritter-Sterr, C., & Miller, D. R. (1987). The measurement of performance in childhood cancer patients. *Cancer, 60,* 1651–1656.

Lovell, D. J., (1992). Newer functional outcome measurements in juvenile rheumatoid arthritis: A progress report. *The Journal of Rheumatology, 19,* 28–31.

Lovell, D. J., Howe, S., Shear, E., Hatner, S., McGirr, G., Schulte, M., & Levinson, J. (1989). Development of a disability measurement tool for juvenile rheumatoid arthritis—the Juvenile Arthritis Functional Assessment Scale. *Arthritis and Rheumatism, 32,* 1390–1395.

Manne, S. L., Redd, W. H., Jacobsen, P. B., Gorfinkle, K., Schorr, O., & Rapkin, B. (1990). Behavioral intervention to reduce child and parent distress during venipuncture. *Journal of Consulting and Clinical Psychology, 58,* 565–572.

Martin, G., & Pear, J. (1999). *Behavior modification: What it is and how to do it* (6th ed.). Upper Saddle River, NJ: Prentice Hall.

Martin, P. R., Milech, D., & Nathan, P. R. (1993). Towards a functional model of chronic headaches: Investigation of antecedents and consequences. *Headache, 33,* 461–470.

Mash, E. J., & Terdal, L. G. (Eds.). (1997). *Assessment of childhood disorders* (3rd ed.). New York: Guilford.

Mattar, M., Martello, J., & Yaffe, S. (1975). Inadequacies in the pharmacologic management of ambulatory children. *Journal of Pediatrics, 87,* 137–141.

McCaul, K. D., & Malott, J. M. (1984). Distraction and coping with pain. *Psychological Bulletin, 95,* 516–533.

McGrath, P. A. (1990). *Pain in children: Nature, assessment, and treatment.* New York: Guilford.

Meichenbaum, D., & Turk, D. C. (1987). *Facilitating treatment adherence: A practitioner's guide.* New York: Plenum.

Melzack, R., & Wall, P. (1965). Pain mechanisms: A new theory. *Science, 150,* 971–979.

Melzack, R. (1993). Pain: Past, present, and future. *Canadian Journal of Experimental Psychology, 47,* 615–629.

Melzack, R., & Wall, P. D. (1982). *The challenge of pain.* New York: Basic Books.

Miller, J. J. (1993). Psychosocial factors related to rheumatic diseases in childhood. *Journal of Rheumatology, 20,* 1–11.

Moos, R. H., Cronkite, R. C., Billings, A. G., & Finney, J. W. (1984). *The Health and Daily Living Form manual.* Social Ecology Laboratory, Stanford University, Stanford, California 94035.

Morse, W. H., & Kelleher, R. T. (1977). Determinants of reinforcement and punishment. In W. K. Honig & J. E. R. Staddon (Eds.), *Handbook of operant behavior* (pp. 174–200). Englewood Cliffs, NJ: Prentice Hall, Inc.

Murray, K. J., & Passo, M. H. (1995). Functional measures in children with rheumatic diseases. *Pediatric Clinics of North America, 42,* 1127–1154.

O'Brien, W. H., & Haynes, S. N. (1995). A functional analytic approach to the conceptualization, assessment and treatment of a child with frequent migraine headaches. *Session: Psychotherapy in Practice, 1,* 65–80.

Ollendick, T. H., & Hersen, M. (Eds.). (1984). *Child behavioral assessment: Principles and procedures.* New York: Pergamon.

Oltmanns, T. F., & Emery, R. E. (1998). *Abnormal psychology* (2nd ed.). New York: Prentice Hall.

Pendley, J. S., Dahlquist, L. M., & Dreyer, Z. (1997). Body image and social adjustment in adolescent cancer survivors. *Journal of Pediatric Psychology, 22,* 29–43.

Pendley, J. S., Dahlquist, L. M., & Cradock, M. M. (August 1996). *Body image and psychosocial adjustment in adolescents with arthritis.* Poster presented at the annual meeting of the American Psychological Association, Toronto, Canada.

Powers, S. W., Blount, R. L., Bachanas, P. J., Cotter, M. W., & Swan, S. C. (1993). Helping preschool leukemia patients and their parents cope during injections. *Journal of Pediatric Psychology, 18,* 681–695.

Rappaport, L., & Frazer, C. H. (1995). Recurrent abdominal pain: Comment. *Journal of Developmental and Behavioral Pediatrics, 16,* 279–281.

Richardson, G. M., McGrath, P. J., Cunningham, S. J., & Humphreys, P. (1983). Validity of the headache diary for children. *Headache, 23,* 184–187.

Ross, D. M., & Ross, S. A. (1988). *Childhood pain: Current issues, research and management.* Baltimore, MD: Urban & Schwarzenberg.

Sacket, D., & Haynes, R. (1976). *Compliance with therapeutic regimens.* Baltimore, MD: Johns Hopkins University Press.

Schechter, N. L. (1989). The undertreatment of pain in children: An overview. *Pediatric Clinics of North America, 36,* 781–794.

Schechter, N. L., Allen, D. A., & Hanson, M. A. (1986). Status of pediatric pain control: A comparison of hospital analgesic usage in children and adults. *Pediatrics, 77*, 11–15.

Sees, K. L., & Clark, H. W. (1993). Opioid use in the treatment of chronic pain: Assessment of addiction. *Journal of Pain and Symptom Management, 8*, 257–264.

Seligman, M. E. P., Maier, S. F., & Solomon, R. L. (1971). Unpredictable and uncontrollable aversive events. In F. R. Bush (Ed.), *Aversive conditioning and learning.* New York: Academic Press.

Singh, G., Athreya, B. H., Fries, J. F., & Goldsmith, D. P. (1994). Measurement of health status in children with juvenile rheumatoid arthritis. *Arthritis and Rheumatism, 37*, 1761–1769.

Sparrow, S., Balla, D., & Cicchetti, D. (1984). *Vineland adpative behavior scales.* Circle Pines, MN: American Guidance Service.

Spielberger, C., Edwards, C., Lushene, R., Monturi, J., & Platzek, S. (1973). *The state-trait anxiety inventory for children.* Palo Alto, CA: Consulting Psychologist Press.

Staub, E., Tursky, B., & Schwartz, G. E. (1971). Self-control and predictability: Their effects on reactions to aversive stimulation. *Journal of Personality and Social Psychology, 18*, 157–162.

Stein, R. E. K., Gortmaker, S. L., Perrin, E. C., Pless, I. B., Walker, D. K., & Weitzman, M. (1987). Severity of illness: Concepts and measurements. *The Lancet, December 26*, 1506–1509.

Stokes, T. F., & Baer, D. M. (1977). An implicit technology of generalization. *Journal of Applied Behavior Analysis, 10*, 349–367.

Switkin, M., & Dahlquist, L. M. (1998). The effects of maternal responsivity and anxiety on child distress during cancer procedures. Unpublished manuscript, University of Maryland Baltimore County.

Thompson, K. L., & Varni, J. W. (1985). A developmental cognitive-biobehavioral approach to pediatric pain assessment. *Pain, 25*, 283–296.

Thompson, S. M., Power, T., & Dahlquist, L. M. (November 1994). *Peer activities and peer networks in children with juvenile rheumatoid arthritis.* Paper presented at the meeting of the Association for the Advancement of Behavior Therapy, San Diego, CA.

Thompson, S. M., Power, T., & Dahlquist, L. M. (1998). Reliability and validity of the Peer Interaction Record: Brief assessment of children's peer activities and companions. Manuscript under review.

Turk, D. C., Meichenbaum, D., & Genest, M. (1983). *Pain and behavioral medicine.* New York: Guilford.

Turk, D. C., & Melzack, R. (Eds.). (1992). *Handbook of pain assessment.* New York: Guilford.

Watson, T. S., & Gresham, F. M. (1998). *Handbook of child behavior therapy.* New York: Plenum.

Weissbluth, M. (1987). *Healthy sleep habits, healthy child.* New York: Fawcett Columbine.

Zabatany, L., Hartman, D. P., & Ranking, D. B. (1990). The psychological functions of preadolescent peer activities. *Child Development, 61*, 1067–1080.

Zeltzer, L. (1995). "Recurrent abdominal pain": Comment. *Journal of Developmental and Behavioral Pediatrics, 16*, 279–281.

Zeltzer, L. K., Barr, R. G., McGrath, P. A., & Schechter, N. L. (1992). Pediatric pain: Interacting behavioral and physical factors. *Pediatrics, 90*, 816–821.

Appendix A

Generating Hypotheses/ Evaluation Planning Worksheet

Hypothesized *physical* contributors	Sources of data	Evaluation plan	Test results
1. Is the child receiving less than optimal pain medication?			
2. Are medications administered inappropriately? • Inappropriate dose? • Inappropriate times? • Inappropriate schedule (p.r.n., breakthrough pain)?			
3. Is the child failing to get all scheduled medication doses? • Adherence problems? • Late or forgotten doses? • Inaccurately measured? • Interfering beliefs/misconceptions?			
4. Are pain medications unavailable?			
5. Are other physical factors exacerbating the child's pain? • Protective posturing? • Muscle tension? • Fatigue? • Environmental factors? • Over-exertion? • PT noncompliance?			

Hypothesized *cognitive/emotional* contributors	Sources of data	Evaluation plan	Test results
1. Is the child's attention focused on the pain?			
2. Is anxiety or stress exacerbating the child's pain?			

3. Does the child engage in self-defeating thinking about the pain?

4. Does the pain have significant meaning for the child?

5. Is the caregiver's emotional or cognitive status interfering?

Hypothesized *behavioral* contributors	Sources of data	Evaluation plan	Test results
1. Is the child's pain behavior positively reinforced?			
2. Is the child's pain behavior negatively reinforced?			
3. Is the child's adaptive behavior inadequately reinforced or punished?			
4. Does the child lack the necessary skills? • Cognitive/academic deficits? • Social/communication deficits? Other?			
5. Is the adult's problematic behavior positively reinforced?			
6. Is the adult's problematic behavior negatively reinforced?			
7. Is appropriate adult behavior inadequately reinforced or punished?			

Appendix B

Treatment Planning Worksheet

Hypothesized *physical* contributors	Test results	Treatment plan
1. Is the child receiving less than optimal pain medication?		
2. Are appropriate medications administered inappropriately? • Inappropriate dose, timing, schedule?		
3. Is the child failing to get all scheduled medication doses? • Adherence problems? • Interfering beliefs/misconceptions		
4. Are pain medications unavailable?		
5. Are other physical factors exacerbating the child's pain? • Protective posturing? • Muscle tension? • Fatigue? • Environmental factors? • Over-exertion? • PT noncompliance?		
Hypothesized *cognitive/emotional* contributors	Test results	Treatment plan
1. Is the child's attention focused on the pain?		
2. Is anxiety or stress exacerbating the child's pain?		
3. Does the child engage in self-defeating thinking about the pain?		
4. Does the pain have significant meaning for the child?		
5. Is the caregiver's emotional or cognitive status interfering?		

Hypothesized *behavioral* contributors	Test results	Treatment plan
1. Is the child's pain behavior positively reinforced?		
2. Is the child's pain behavior negatively reinforced?		
3. Is adaptive behavior inadequately reinforced or punished?		
4. Does the child lack the skills necessary to perform the adaptive behavior? • Cognitive/academic deficits? • Social/communication deficits? • Other		
5. To what degree is the adult's problematic behavior positively reinforced?		
6. To what degree is the adult's problematic behavior negatively reinforced?		
7. Is appropriate adult behavior inadequately reinforced or punished?		

Peer Interaction Record (PIR)

PIR Child Report (Administer via Interview) (Rev 3/20/98)

Number _____ Name _____ Age _____ Date: _____

Interviewer_____

In the past week (past 7 days), how often did you do the following activities with FRIENDS (not family members)?

		Yes or no	If yes, how many times last week?	With whom did you do it? List first names	Is this person a boy or a girl? (Circle one)		How old is this friend?
1.	Did you eat a meal with a friend (other than at school)?				Boy	Girl	
					Boy	Girl	
					Boy	Girl	
					Boy	Girl	
					Boy	Girl	
2.	Did you watch TV or listen to music with a friend?				Boy	Girl	
					Boy	Girl	
					Boy	Girl	
					Boy	Girl	
					Boy	Girl	
3.	Did you work on homework or a school project with a friend (when not at school)?				Boy	Girl	
					Boy	Girl	
					Boy	Girl	
					Boy	Girl	
					Boy	Girl	

		Yes or no	If yes, how many times last week?	With whom did you do it? List first names	Is this person a boy or a girl? (Circle one)		How old is this friend?
4.	Did you have a friend over?				Boy	Girl	
					Boy	Girl	
					Boy	Girl	
					Boy	Girl	
					Boy	Girl	
5.	Did you go to a friend's house?				Boy	Girl	
					Boy	Girl	
					Boy	Girl	
					Boy	Girl	
					Boy	Girl	
6.	Did you go to a club meeting (e.g., scouts, YMCA, church club, 4H)?			NA	Boys only		How old are the other children in the club? List ages:
					Girls only		
					Boys and girls		
7.	Did you play a team sport with an adult coach after school or on the weekend (e.g., swim team, baseball, gymnastics, soccer, tennis)?			NA	Boys only		How old are the other children on the team? List ages:
					Girls only		
					Boys and girls		
8.	Did you go somewhere with a friend, like to the movies, the beach, skating?				Boy	Girl	
					Boy	Girl	
					Boy	Girl	
					Boy	Girl	
					Boy	Girl	
9.	Did you go to a friend's party?			NA	Boys only		How old were the other children at the party? List ages:
					Girls only		
					Boys and girls		

		Yes or no	If yes, how many times last week?	With whom did you do it? List first names	Is this person a boy or a girl? (Circle one)		How old is this friend?
10.	Did you go shopping or go to the mall with a friend?				Boy	Girl	
					Boy	Girl	
					Boy	Girl	
					Boy	Girl	
					Boy	Girl	
11.	Did you play an outdoor game or activity with a friend (e.g., softball, swimming)?				Boy	Girl	
					Boy	Girl	
					Boy	Girl	
					Boy	Girl	
					Boy	Girl	
12.	Did you play an indoor game or activity with a friend (e.g., computer game, cards, board game, crafts)?				Boy	Girl	
					Boy	Girl	
					Boy	Girl	
					Boy	Girl	
					Boy	Girl	
					Boy	Girl	
13.	Who are your friends? List first name, whether the friend is a boy or girl, and the friend's age.	First name			Boy or girl		Age

PIR Parent Report (Administer via interview) (rev 3/20/98)

Number _____ Name_____ Age _____ Date: _____
Interviewer_____

In the past week (past 7 days), how often did your child do the following activities with FRIENDS (not family members)?						

		Yes or no	If yes, how many times last week?	With whom did your child do it? List first names	Is this person a boy or a girl? (Circle one)		How old is this friend?
1.	Did your child eat a meal with a friend (other than at school)?				Boy	Girl	
					Boy	Girl	
					Boy	Girl	
					Boy	Girl	
					Boy	Girl	
2.	Did your child watch TV or listen to music with a friend?				Boy	Girl	
					Boy	Girl	
					Boy	Girl	
					Boy	Girl	
					Boy	Girl	
3.	Did your child work on homework or a school project with a friend (when not at school)?				Boy	Girl	
					Boy	Girl	
					Boy	Girl	
					Boy	Girl	
					Boy	Girl	
4.	Did your child have a friend over?				Boy	Girl	
					Boy	Girl	
					Boy	Girl	
					Boy	Girl	
					Boy	Girl	

		Yes or no	If yes, how many times last week?	With whom did your child do it? List first names	Is this person a boy or a girl? (Circle one)		How old is this friend?
5.	Did your child go to a friend's house?				Boy	Girl	
					Boy	Girl	
					Boy	Girl	
					Boy	Girl	
					Boy	Girl	
6.	Did your child go to a club meeting (e.g., scouts, YMCA, church club, 4H)?			NA	Boys only		How old are the other children in the club? List ages:
					Girls only		
					Boys and girls		
7.	Did your child play a team sport with an adult coach after school or on the weekend (e.g., swim team, baseball, gymnastics, soccer, tennis)?			NA	Boys only		How old are the other children on the team? List ages:
					Girls only		
					Boys and girls		
8.	Did your child go somewhere with a friend, like to the movies, the beach, skating?				Boy	Girl	
					Boy	Girl	
					Boy	Girl	
					Boy	Girl	
					Boy	Girl	
9.	Did your child go to a friend's party?			NA	Boys only		How old were the other children at the party? List ages:
					Girls only		
					Boys and girls		

		Yes or no	If yes, how many times last week?	With whom did your child do it? List first names	Is this person a boy or a girl? (Circle one)		How old is this friend?
10.	Did your child go shopping or go to the mall with a friend?				Boy	Girl	
					Boy	Girl	
					Boy	Girl	
					Boy	Girl	
					Boy	Girl	
11.	Did your child play an outdoor game or activity with a friend (e.g., softball, swimming)?				Boy	Girl	
					Boy	Girl	
					Boy	Girl	
					Boy	Girl	
					Boy	Girl	
12.	Did your child play an indoor game or activity with a friend (e.g., computer game, cards, board game, crafts)?				Boy	Girl	
					Boy	Girl	
					Boy	Girl	
					Boy	Girl	
					Boy	Girl	
13.	Who are your child's friends? List first name, whether the friend is a boy or girl, and the friend's age.	First name			Boy or girl		Age

Appendix D

Selected Readings

GENERAL READINGS ON PAIN IN CHILDREN

Bush, J. P., & Harkins, S. W. (1991). *Children in pain: Clinical and research issues from a developmental perspective.* New York: Springer Verlag.

Bush, J. P., Holmbeck, G. N., & Cockrelli, J. L. (1989). Patterns of PRN analgesic drug administration in children following elective surgery. *Journal of Pediatric Psychology, 14*, 433–448.

Ross, D. M., & Ross, S. A. (1988). *Childhood pain: Current issues, research and management.* Baltimore, MD: Urban & Schwarzenberg.

McGrath, P. A. (1990). *Pain in children: Nature, assessment, and treatment.* New York: Guilford.

Schechter, N. (1989). The undertreatment of pain in children: An overview. *Pediatric Clinics of North America, 36*, 781–794.

Zeltzer, L. K., Barr, R. G., McGrath, P. A., & Schechter, N. L. (1992). Pediatric pain: Interacting behavioral and physical factors. *Pediatrics, 90*, 816–821.

PAIN MEDICATIONS

Acute Pain Management Guideline Panel. (February 1992). *Acute pain management: Operative or medical procedures and trauma. Clinical practice guideline.* AHCPR Pub. No. 92-0032. Rockville, MD: Agency for Health Care Policy and Research, Public Health Service, U.S. Department of Health and Human Services. (To order this publication and related *Guideline Report* and *Quick Reference Guide for Clinicians* call the AHCPR Clearinghouse at (800)358-9295 or write to the Center for Research Dissemination and Liaison, AHCPR Clearinghouse, P.O. Box 8547, Silver Spring, MD 20907.)

ADHERENCE TO MEDICATION REGIMENS

Meichenbaum, D., & Turk, D. C. (1987). *Facilitating treatment adherence: A practitioner's guide.* New York: Plenum.

RECURRENT AND CHRONIC PAIN ─────────────────────────────────

Allen, K. D., & Matthews, J. R. (1998). Behavior management of recurrent pain in children. In T. S. Watson & F. M. Gresham (Eds.), *Handbook of child behavior therapy* (pp. 263–285). New York: Plenum.

Barlow, C. F. (1984). *Headaches and migraine in childhood*. Philadelphia: J. B. Lippincott.

Fordyce, W. E. (1976). *Behavioral methods for chronic pain and illness*. St. Louis, MO: Mosby.

Novy, D. M., Nelson, D. V., Francis, D. J., & Turk, D. C. (1995). Perspectives of chronic pain: An evaluative comparison of restrictive and comprehensive models. *Psychological Bulletin, 118,* 238–247.

Scharff, L. (1997). Recurrent abdominal pain in children: A review of psychological factors and treatment. *Clinical Psychology Review, 17,* 145–166.

Wilson, J. J., & Gil, K. M. (1996). The efficacy of psychological and pharmacological interventions for the treatment of chronic disease-related and non-disease-related pain. *Clinical Psychology Review, 16,* 573–597.

PAIN QUESTIONNAIRES FOR CHILDREN ─────────────────────────

McGrath, P. A. (1990). *Pain in children: Nature, assessment, and treatment*. New York: Guilford.

Varni, J. W., & Thompson, K. L. (1985). The Varni/Thompson Pediatric Pain Questionnaire. Unpublished manuscript.

Varni, J. W., Waldron, S. A., Gragg, R. A., Rapoff, M. A., Bernstein, B. H., Lindsley, C. B., & Newcomb, M. D. (1996). The Waldron/Varni Pediatric Pain Coping Inventory. Unpublished manuscript.[*]

CONSULTATION WITH MEDICAL PROFESSIONALS ────────────────

Drotar, D. (1995). *Consulting with pediatricians: Psychological perspectives*. New York: Plenum.

BIOFEEDBACK ───

Schwartz, M. S. (Ed.). (1995). *Biofeedback: A practitioner's guide* (2nd ed.). New York: Guilford.

SOCIAL SKILLS, SOCIAL ADJUSTMENT ─────────────────────────

Gresham, F. M. (1998). Social skills training with children: Social learning and behavioral analytic approaches. In T. S. Watson & F. M. Gresham (Eds.). (1998). *Handbook of child behavior therapy* (pp. 475–498). New York: Plenum.

---

[*] Copies of the Varni et al. Scales can be obtained from James Varni, Ph.D., Psychosocial & Behavioral Sciences Program, Division of Hematology-Oncology, Children's Hospital and Health Center, 3020 Children's Way MOB #103, San Diego, CA 92123-4282.

Rubin, K., & Stewart, S. L. (1996). Social withdrawal. In E. J. Mash & R. A. Barkley (Eds.), *Child psychopathology* (pp. 277–307). New York: Guilford.

Hops, H. (1988). Social skills deficits. In E. J. Mash & L. G. Terdal (Eds.), *Behavioral assessment of childhood disorders* (2nd ed., pp. 263–314). New York: Guilford.

Albano, A. M., Chorpita, B. F., & Barlow, D. H. (1996). Childhood anxiety disorders. In E. J. Mash & R. A. Barkley (Eds.), *Child psychopathology* (pp. 196–241). New York: Guilford.

ASSESSMENT OF COMMON CLINICAL PROBLEMS IN CHILDREN

Mash, E. J., & Terdal, L. G. (Eds.). (1997). *Assessment of childhood disorders* (3rd ed.). New York: Guilford. (Text includes chapters on conduct disorders, depression, fears and anxiety, learning disability, family conflict and communication.)

LaGreca, A. M. (Ed.). (1990). *Through the eyes of the child: Obtaining child reports from children and adolescents*. New York: Allyn & Bacon.

Schroeder, C. S., & Gordon, B. N. (1991). *Assessment and treatment of childhood problems: A clinician's guide*. New York: Guilford.

BEHAVIORAL ASSESSMENT AND BEHAVIOR THERAPY

Gross, A. M. (1984). Behavioral interviewing. In T. H. Ollendick & M. Hersen (Eds.), *Child Behavioral assessment: Principles and procedures* (pp. 61–79). New York: Pergamon.

O'Brien, W. H., & Haynes, S. N. (1995). A functional analytic approach to the conceptualization, assessment and treatment of a child with frequent migraine headaches. *In Session: Psychotherapy in Practice, 1,* 65–80.

Ollendick, T. H., & Hersen, M. (Eds.) (1984). *Child behavioral assessment: Principles and procedures* (pp. 61–79). New York: Pergamon.

Martin, G., & Pear, J. (1999). *Behavior modification: What it is and how to do it* (5th ed.). Upper Saddle River, NJ: Prentice-Hall.

Watson, T. S., & Gresham, F. M. (Eds.). (1998). *Handbook of child behavior therapy*. New York: Plenum.

Index